BEAT CANCER, THE ANTI CANCER KITCHEN

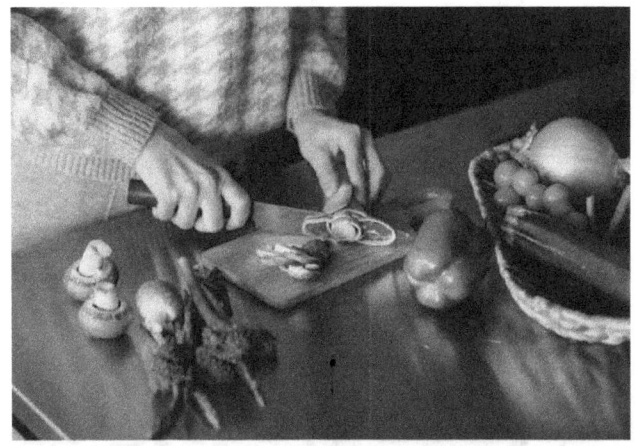

Transforming Your Kitchen Into A Weapon Against Cancer

Raquel Williams

Copyright © 2024 by Raquel Williams

All rights reserved. This book or any portion thereof may not be reproduced or used in any manner whatsoever without the express written permission of the author except for the use of brief quotations in a book review.

My Author Central page

INTRODUCTION

Welcome to "Beat Cancer, The Anti-Cancer Kitchen," where the power of nutrition becomes your greatest ally in the fight against cancer. In this transformative guide, you will unveil a treasure trove of cancer-fighting recipes and plant-based nutrition strategies designed to empower you on your journey to wellness.

Harnessing the healing potential of nutrient-rich meals, this book is not just about food, it's about adopting a holistic approach to health through the ingredients that grace your kitchen. From the therapeutic benefits of healing herbs and spices to the immune-boosting properties of superfoods, each recipe is meticulously crafted to nourish your body and fortify your spirit.

Join as I explore the intersection of culinary artistry and science-backed nutrition, revealing how simple lifestyle changes can yield profound results in cancer prevention and recovery. With a focus on anti-inflammatory foods and integrative medicine principles, you'll discover the transformative power of wholesome ingredients in combating cancer and promoting overall wellness. Whether you're seeking preventive measures or navigating the path to recovery, "Beat Cancer, The Anti-Cancer Kitchen" offers a roadmap to resilience, empowering you to take control of your health and embrace a life of vitality. It's time to embark on a journey of healing, one delicious bite at a time.

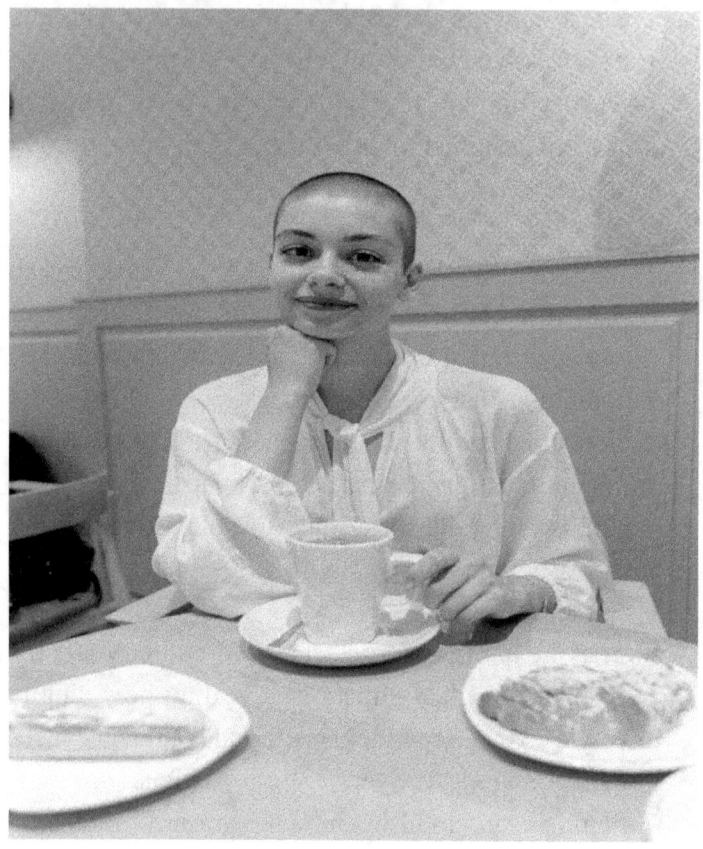

TABLE OF CONTENTS

INTRODUCTION   2
TABLE OF CONTENTS   5
Getting Started   8
    Understanding the Battle Against Cancer   11
    The Role of Diet in Cancer Prevention   11
    How to Use This Book   15
    A Note from the Author   17
Chapter 1: The Science of Cancer and Nutrition
    Understanding Cancer, Causes and Mechanisms   19
    The Link Between Diet and Cancer   21
    Key Anticancer Nutrients   25
    Scientific Studies and Evidence   27
Chapter 2: Stocking Your Anticancer Kitchen   31
    Essential Anti-Cancer Foods   31
    Organising Your Pantry   33
    Shopping Tips for Anti-Cancer Ingredients   36
    Tools and Gadgets for a Healthy Kitchen   39
Chapter 3: Superfoods That Fight Cancer   43
    The Power of Berries and Fruits   43
    Cruciferous Vegetables, A Potent Ally   46
    Whole Grains and Legumes   50
    Spices and Herbs with Anti-Cancer Properties
Chapter 4: Anti-Cancer Breakfasts   57
    Energising Smoothies   57
    Nutrient-Packed Oatmeals   60
    Anti-Cancer Breakfast Bowls   64
    Healthy Morning Beverages   67

Chapter 5: Immune-Boosting Lunches 71
   Superfood Salads 71
   Nutritious Grain Bowls 74
   Hearty Soups and Stews 76
   Anti-Cancer Sandwiches and Wraps 78
Chapter 6: Delicious and Healthy Dinners 83
   Plant-Based Main Courses 83
   Lean Proteins and Fish Recipes 86
   Cancer-Fighting Side Dishes 88
   Balanced Dinner Plates 92
Chapter 7: Snacks and Small Bites 95
   Quick and Healthy Snacks 95
   Anti-Cancer Dips and Spreads 98
   Nutritious Bars and Bites 101
   Portable Snacks for On-the-Go 104
Chapter 8: Desserts with Benefits 107
   Guilt-Free Sweet Treats 107
   Anti-Cancer Baking 109
   Fruit-Based Desserts 112
   Indulgent Yet Healthy Puddings 115
Chapter 9: Beverages That Heal 119
   Anti-Inflammatory Teas 119
   Detoxifying Juices 122
   Smoothies for Health 125
   Hydrating and Healing Drinks 128
Chapter 10: Meal Planning and Preparation 131
   Creating an Anti-Cancer Meal Plan 131
   Batch Cooking and Freezing Tips 134
   Balancing Nutrients Throughout the Day 137
   Sample Weekly Menus 139

Chapter 11: Dining Out and Social Events   143
    Making Smart Choices at Restaurants   143
    Navigating Social Gatherings   146
    Bringing Your Own Anticancer Dishes   149
Chapter 12: The Mind-Body Connection   155
    Stress Management and Cancer Prevention 155
    Incorporating Mindfulness into Meals   158
    Physical Activity and Nutrition   161
    Sleep and Recovery   167
Chapter 13: Real-Life Success Stories   172
    Inspiring Journeys of Cancer Survivors   173
    How Diet Made a Difference   176
    Practical Tips from Real People   179
    Lessons Learned and Hope for the Future   182
Chapter 14: Special Considerations   185
    Diet and Cancer Treatment Side Effects   185
    Adjusting Your Diet Post-Diagnosis   188
    Anti-Cancer Diets for Different Age Groups   193
    Addressing Common Nutritional Deficiencies
Chapter 15: Moving Forward   204
    Sustaining an Anti-Cancer Lifestyle   204
    Continuous Learning and Adaptation   208
    Building a Support System   211
    Final Thoughts and Encouragement   215
CONCLUSION   219
Free special Bonus for you   222

Getting Started

Getting started on your journey to creating an anti-cancer kitchen involves incorporating foods and recipes that are rich in nutrients, antioxidants, and anti-inflammatory properties. Begin by stocking your kitchen with fresh fruits, vegetables, herbs, spices, nuts, seeds, legumes, and whole grains these are the building blocks of an anticancer diet.

1. Introduction to the book's theme: Understanding the Battle Against Cancer" this sets the stage by introducing readers to the central theme of combating cancer through dietary changes. It highlights the importance of nutrition in cancer prevention and management.

2. Foundational understanding of cancer: This chapter provides readers with a foundational understanding of cancer, including its biological mechanisms and how it develops. It may cover topics such as cell growth, mutations, and tumour formation.

3. Exploration of nutrition's role: Readers should learn about the significant role that nutrition plays in cancer prevention and management. The chapter may discuss how certain dietary patterns and food choices can impact cancer risk and progression.

4. Basic biology of cancer: Delving deeper, this section explains the basic biology of cancer, including how cancer cells differ from healthy cells and how tumours grow and spread throughout the body.

5. Common risk factors: Readers gain insight into common risk factors associated with cancer, such as smoking, poor diet, lack of physical activity, exposure to carcinogens, and genetic predisposition.

6. Importance of early detection: The chapter emphasises the importance of early detection and diagnosis in improving cancer outcomes. It may discuss screening tests and the benefits of detecting cancer at an early stage when treatment is most effective.

7. Emotional and psychological aspects: Recognizing the emotional and psychological impact of a cancer diagnosis, this section addresses coping strategies and support systems available to individuals and their loved ones facing cancer.

8. Setting the stage for practical advice: While laying the groundwork for the practical advice and guidance offered in subsequent chapters, this section prepares readers for the transformative journey they will embark on in their kitchen.

9. Preparation for the kitchen journey: Readers are motivated and empowered to take proactive steps in their health journey, understanding that their kitchen can be a powerful tool in the fight against cancer.

10. Understanding lifestyle choices: This chapter highlights the link between lifestyle choices, including diet, and cancer risk, encouraging readers to make informed decisions about their health habits.

11. Empowerment to make informed choices: Through education and understanding, readers are empowered to make informed decisions about their health and lifestyle, recognizing the impact these choices can have on cancer risk and overall well-being.

12. Encouragement for proactive prevention: The chapter encourages readers to adopt a proactive approach to cancer prevention, emphasising the importance of taking control of one's health through dietary and lifestyle changes.

Understanding the Battle Against Cancer

Understanding the Battle Against Cancer" serves as the opening chapter of the book, readers should embark on their journey toward understanding and combating cancer through nutrition. This chapter introduces readers to the overarching theme of the book and aims to provide them with a foundational understanding of cancer, its causes, and the role that nutrition plays in prevention and management.

It may delve into the basic biology of cancer, common risk factors, and the importance of early detection. Additionally, it might touch upon the emotional and psychological aspects of coping with a cancer diagnosis, setting the stage for the practical advice and guidance that follows in subsequent chapters. Overall, this chapter serves as a primer for readers, laying the groundwork for the transformative journey they are about to embark on in their kitchen.

The Role of Diet in Cancer Prevention

Diet plays a crucial role in cancer prevention, as the food we eat directly affects our bodies' overall health and ability to fight off diseases. Research has shown that certain dietary patterns and specific foods can help reduce the risk of developing cancer.

1. Nutrient Intake: A balanced diet rich in essential nutrients like vitamins, minerals, antioxidants, and fibre supports the body's immune system and overall health, helping to prevent cellular damage and reduce the risk of cancer development.

2. Weight Management: Maintaining a healthy weight through a combination of proper diet and regular physical activity is crucial for cancer prevention. Excess body weight, particularly obesity, is associated with an increased risk of several types of cancer, including breast, colorectal, and prostate cancer.

3. Reducing Inflammation: Chronic inflammation in the body is linked to an increased risk of cancer. Certain foods, such as fruits, vegetables, and omega-3 fatty acids found in fish, help reduce inflammation and lower cancer risk.

4. Antioxidant Protection: Antioxidants found in fruits, vegetables, and other plant-based foods help neutralise harmful free radicals in the body, which can damage cells and contribute to cancer development. Including a variety of colourful fruits and vegetables in the diet ensures an adequate intake of antioxidants.

5. Healthy Gut Microbiota: The balance of bacteria in the gut, known as the gut microbiota, plays a crucial role in maintaining immune function and protecting against cancer. A diet rich in fibre, prebiotics, and probiotics promotes a diverse and healthy gut microbiota, reducing inflammation and lowering the risk of gastrointestinal cancers.

6. Limiting Carcinogens: Certain dietary factors, such as excessive consumption of processed meats, charred meats, and foods high in saturated fats, have been linked to an increased risk of cancer. Limiting exposure to these carcinogens can help lower cancer risk.

7. Hydration: Staying hydrated is essential for overall health and can help prevent cancer by supporting proper cellular function and detoxification processes. Drinking plenty of water and consuming hydrating foods like fruits and vegetables can help maintain hydration levels and reduce cancer risk.

8. Lifestyle Factors: Adopting a holistic approach to health, including regular physical activity, avoiding tobacco, limiting alcohol consumption, and managing stress, significantly reduces cancer risk by addressing multiple lifestyle factors that contribute to overall health and wellbeing.

9. Balancing Macronutrients: A balanced diet that includes a mix of carbohydrates, proteins, and healthy fats provides the body with the energy and nutrients it needs to function optimally, supporting immune function and reducing cancer risk.

10. Moderating Sugar and Refined Carbohydrates: Excessive consumption of sugar and refined carbohydrates can contribute to weight gain and inflammation, increasing the risk of cancer. Moderating intake of sugary snacks and processed foods helps control blood sugar levels and reduces cancer risk.

11. Including Phytochemicals: Phytochemicals are natural compounds found in plant foods that have protective effects against cancer. Including a variety of fruits, vegetables, herbs, and spices in the diet ensures a diverse intake of phytochemicals, which can help reduce inflammation, regulate cell growth, and inhibit cancer development.

12. Promoting Immune Function: Nutrient-rich foods support immune function, helping the body identify and eliminate cancerous cells before they can develop into tumours. A diet rich in fruits, vegetables, nuts, and seeds provides vitamins, minerals, and antioxidants that support immune function and help prevent cancer.

How to Use This Book

This book section serves as a guide for readers on navigating the content and making the most out of the information provided. Here's how it could be structured.

1. Introduction: Begin by welcoming readers and providing an overview of the book's purpose and contents. Explain that the section aims to help readers maximize their experience and benefit from the information presented.

2. Navigating Chapters: Provide a brief overview of the book's structure and chapters. Highlight the progression of topics from understanding cancer and nutrition to practical tips for incorporating cancer-fighting foods into everyday meals.

3. Setting Goals: readers should set personal goals for their health journey based on the information presented in the book. Whether it's adopting healthier eating habits, managing weight, or reducing cancer risk factors, setting clear goals can help readers stay focused and motivated.

4. **Interactive Features:** Highlight any interactive features or tools included in the book, such as meal planning templates, shopping lists, or journaling prompts. readers should actively engage with these features to enhance their learning experience.

5. **Action Steps:** Provide actionable steps or challenges at the end of each chapter to encourage readers to apply the information to their daily lives. These could include trying new recipes, incorporating specific foods into their diet, or setting short-term health goals.

6. **Tracking Progress:** readers should track their progress and achievements throughout their health journey. Whether it's keeping a food diary, monitoring physical activity, or tracking changes in health metrics, tracking progress can help readers stay accountable and motivated.

7. **Seeking Support:** readers should remember that they are not alone on their health journey. Seek support from friends, family, or healthcare professionals as needed. Provide resources or references for additional support, such as support

groups, online forums, or healthcare providers specialising in nutrition and cancer prevention.

8. **Conclusion:** Conclude the section by reinforcing the importance of taking an active role in one's health and using the information provided in the book as a tool for empowerment and transformation.

A Note from the Author

Welcome to "Beat Cancer, the Anti-Cancer Kitchen," where the transformative potential of nutrition meets the power of your kitchen.

As the author of this book, I'm honoured to join you on this journey towards optimal health and vitality. My personal battle against cancer ignited a passion for nutrition, leading me to compile this comprehensive guide to empower you in your own fight against cancer.

Within these pages, you'll uncover evidence-based insights, practical tips, and tantalising recipes meticulously crafted to nourish your body and fortify your immune system. From understanding the science behind cancer and nutrition to stocking your kitchen with anti-cancer essentials, each chapter is tailored to equip you with the knowledge and tools necessary to reclaim control of your health.

Yet, amidst the recipes and meal plans lies a beacon of hope, an invitation to not merely survive, but to thrive. With each nutrient-rich meal and mindful lifestyle choice, you're not just combating a disease; you're embracing a life brimming with vitality and purpose.

So, dear reader, as you embark on this transformative journey, know that you're not alone. I'm here to walk alongside with you, offering guidance, support, and unwavering encouragement. Together, let's unlock the healing potential of nutrition, cultivate resilience, and redefine what it means to thrive in the face of adversity.

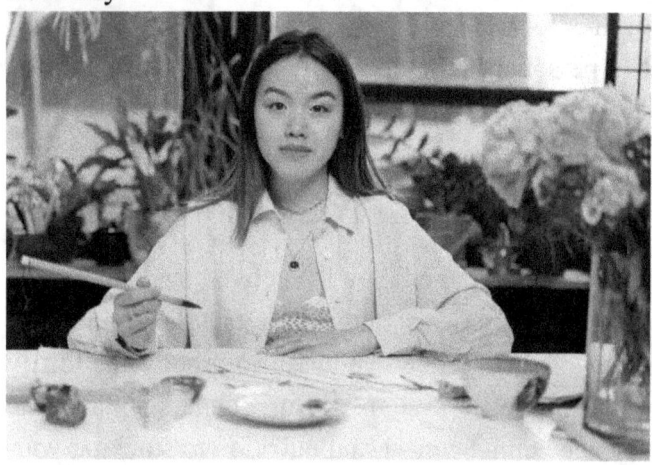

Chapter 1: The Science of Cancer and Nutrition

Understanding Cancer, Causes and Mechanisms

Understanding Cancer, Causes and Mechanisms serves as a foundational chapter in "Beat Cancer, the Anti Cancer Kitchen," delving into the intricate complexities of cancer development. Here's how it could be structured.

1. Cancer Basics: Provide a primer on cancer, explaining that it is a group of diseases characterised by the abnormal growth and spread of cells. Define key terms such as tumour, metastasis, and carcinogenesis to lay the groundwork for further exploration.

3. Causes of Cancer: Explore the various factors that contribute to the development of cancer, including genetic mutations, environmental exposures, lifestyle choices, and infectious agents. Discuss how these factors can interact and contribute to the initiation and progression of cancer.

4. Mechanisms of Cancer: Dive into the biological mechanisms underlying cancer development, including uncontrolled cell growth, genetic mutations, angiogenesis, and evasion of immune surveillance. Explain how these processes contribute to tumour formation and progression.

5. Risk Factor: Identify common risk factors associated with cancer, such as age, family history, tobacco use, excessive alcohol consumption, poor diet, obesity, and exposure to carcinogens. Discuss how these risk factors can influence cancer development and the importance of risk reduction strategies.

6. Types of Cancer: Provide an overview of the different types of cancer, categorizing them based on their origin (e.g., breast cancer, lung cancer, colon cancer) and highlighting their unique characteristics and risk factors.

7. Prevention Strategies: Offer practical tips and strategies for cancer prevention, including adopting a healthy lifestyle, maintaining a balanced diet, avoiding tobacco and excessive alcohol consumption, practising sun safety, and undergoing regular screenings.

8. Hormonal Factors: Discuss how hormonal imbalances, such as those seen in hormone-related cancers like breast and prostate cancer, can contribute to cancer development.

9. Immune System Dysfunction: Examine how dysregulation of the immune system can allow cancer cells to evade detection and destruction.

10. Epigenetic Changes: Explore how alterations in gene expression patterns, known as epigenetic changes, can influence cancer development.

11. Metabolic Factors: Discuss the role of metabolic dysregulation in cancer growth and progression, including the Warburg effect and altered nutrient metabolism.

12. Microenvironment Influence: Investigate how the tumour microenvironment, including factors like hypoxia and angiogenesis, can promote cancer growth and metastasis.

The Link Between Diet and Cancer

the link between diet and cancer is a critical endeavor in understanding how our food choices can impact our health. Here's a structured outline to delve into this important topic.

1. Diet and Cancer: Set the stage by highlighting the significance of diet in cancer prevention and treatment. Emphasise that dietary factors play a substantial role in modulating cancer risk and progression.

2. Epidemiological Evidence: Discuss findings from epidemiological studies that have investigated the relationship between diet and cancer risk. Highlight key studies and their implications for understanding dietary influences on cancer incidence.

3. Carcinogenic Substances: Explore how certain dietary components, such as processed meats, charred meats, and foods high in saturated fats, can contain carcinogenic substances that contribute to cancer development. Discuss the importance of limiting exposure to these substances.

4. Antioxidants and Phytochemicals: Examine the protective effects of antioxidants and phytochemicals found in fruits, vegetables, herbs, and spices. Discuss how these compounds help neutralise free radicals, reduce inflammation, and inhibit cancer cell growth.

5. Fibre and Gut Health: Investigate the role of dietary fibre in promoting gut health and reducing the risk of colorectal cancer. Discuss how fiber helps regulate bowel movements, maintain a healthy microbiome, and prevent the development of cancerous lesions.

6. Nutrient Density and Cancer Prevention: Highlight the importance of consuming nutrient-dense foods, such as fruits, vegetables, whole grains, and lean proteins, in reducing cancer risk. Discuss how these foods provide essential vitamins, minerals, and antioxidants that support overall health and bolster the immune system.

7. Glycemic Index and Cancer Risk: Explore the impact of high-glycemic-index foods on cancer risk, particularly in relation to insulin resistance, inflammation, and tumour growth. Discuss the benefits of choosing low-glycemic-index foods to help regulate blood sugar levels and reduce cancer risk.

8. Alcohol Consumption: Examine the relationship between alcohol consumption and cancer risk, particularly for cancers of the breast, liver, oesophagus, and colon. Discuss the mechanisms by which alcohol can increase cancer risk and the importance of moderation or abstinence.

9. Processed Foods and Additives: Discuss the potential carcinogenic effects of certain additives and preservatives found in processed foods. Highlight the importance of choosing whole, minimally processed foods to reduce exposure to these harmful substances.

10. **Role of Obesity:** Explore how obesity, often influenced by dietary factors, can increase the risk of several cancers, including breast, colorectal, and prostate cancer. Discuss the importance of maintaining a healthy weight through balanced nutrition and regular physical activity.

11. **Healthy Eating Patterns:** Discuss the benefits of adopting healthy eating patterns, such as the Mediterranean diet or the DASH (Dietary Approaches to Stop Hypertension) diet, in reducing cancer risk. Highlight the emphasis on whole foods, plant-based nutrition, and moderation of red and processed meats.

12. **Recommendations:** Summarise key findings and recommendations for optimising dietary choices to reduce cancer risk. Encourage readers to prioritise a diet rich in fruits, vegetables, whole grains, and lean proteins while minimising intake of processed and sugary foods.

Key Anticancer Nutrients

Understanding the key nutrients that play a role in cancer prevention is essential for making informed dietary choices. Here's how to explore this topic.

1. **Anti-Cancer Nutrients:** Set the stage by emphasising the importance of specific nutrients in reducing cancer risk and supporting overall health.

2. **Vitamins:** Discuss the role of vitamins, such as vitamin A, vitamin C, vitamin D, and vitamin E, in protecting cells from oxidative damage, boosting the immune system, and regulating cell growth and differentiation.

3. **Minerals:** Explore the significance of minerals like selenium, zinc, calcium, and magnesium in maintaining cellular function, DNA repair, and immune response, all of which contribute to cancer prevention.

4. **Antioxidants:** Highlight the importance of antioxidants, such as beta-carotene, lycopene, and flavonoids, in neutralising free radicals and reducing oxidative stress, which can contribute to cancer development.

5. Omega-3 Fatty Acids: Discuss the anti-inflammatory properties of omega-3 fatty acids found in fatty fish, flaxseeds, and walnuts, and their potential role in reducing the risk of certain cancers, such as breast and colon cancer.

6. Fibre: Examine the benefits of dietary fibre in promoting digestive health, regulating blood sugar levels, and reducing the risk of colorectal cancer. Discuss sources of fibre-rich foods, such as fruits, vegetables, whole grains, and legumes.

7. Phytochemicals: Explore the diverse array of phytochemicals found in plant foods, such as carotenoids, polyphenols, and glucosinolates, and their potential anti-cancer properties, including antioxidant, anti-inflammatory, and anti-proliferative effects.

8. Probiotics and Prebiotics: Discuss the role of probiotics and prebiotics in promoting a healthy gut microbiota, which can in turn support immune function and reduce the risk of gastrointestinal cancers.

9. Isoflavones and Lignans: Examine the potential cancer-protective effects of isoflavones found in soybeans and lignans found in flaxseeds, which have been linked to reduced risk of hormone-related cancers, such as breast and prostate cancer.

10. Curcumin: Highlight the anti-inflammatory and antioxidant properties of curcumin, the active compound in turmeric, and its potential role in cancer prevention and treatment.

11. Resveratrol: Discuss the health benefits of resveratrol, a polyphenol found in red wine, grapes, and berries, and its potential anti-cancer effects, including inhibition of tumour growth and promotion of apoptosis.

12. Recommendations: Summarise key anticancer nutrients and their sources, and provide practical recommendations for incorporating these nutrients into a balanced diet to reduce cancer risk and support overall health.

Scientific Studies and Evidence

studies and evidence regarding the link between diet and cancer is crucial for understanding the validity of dietary recommendations. Here's how to approach this topic.

1. Scientific Studies: Begin by emphasising the importance of evidence-based research in understanding the relationship between diet and cancer. Highlight the role of scientific studies in providing insights into causation, correlation, and potential mechanisms.

2. **Epidemiological Studies:** Discuss the findings of epidemiological studies that have investigated dietary patterns and cancer incidence among different populations. Highlight key studies and their contributions to our understanding of the relationship between diet and cancer risk.

3. **Clinical Trials:** Explore the results of clinical trials that have examined the effects of specific dietary interventions, such as supplementation with vitamins, minerals, or phytochemicals, on cancer prevention or treatment outcomes.

4. **Mechanistic Studies:** Examine mechanistic studies that have investigated the biological mechanisms underlying the observed effects of dietary factors on cancer development and progression. Discuss how these studies help elucidate the pathways through which diet may influence cancer risk.

5. **Meta-Analyses and Systematic Reviews:** Highlight the findings of meta-analyses and systematic reviews that have synthesised data from

multiple studies to provide a comprehensive overview of the evidence linking diet to cancer risk. Discuss the strengths and limitations of these analyses and their implications for public health recommendations.

6. Biomarker Studies: Discuss the use of biomarkers, such as circulating levels of nutrients or markers of inflammation, in assessing the impact of diet on cancer risk. Explore studies that have examined biomarker profiles in relation to dietary patterns and cancer outcomes.

7. Longitudinal Studies: Examine longitudinal studies that have followed individuals over time to assess the association between diet and cancer incidence or mortality. Discuss how these studies provide valuable insights into the long-term effects of dietary habits on cancer risk.

8. Animal Studies: Explore findings from animal studies that have investigated the effects of specific dietary components or interventions on cancer development in experimental models.

9. Critique of Evidence: Provide a critical analysis of the strengths and limitations of the existing evidence linking diet to cancer risk. Discuss factors such as study design, sample size, confounding variables, and generalizability that may influence the interpretation of study findings.

10. Nutritional Cohort Studies: Discuss the findings of large-scale cohort studies that have followed participants over an extended period to investigate the association between dietary intake and cancer risk. Explore how these studies account for confounding variables and provide valuable insights into the long-term effects of diet on cancer incidence.

11. Dose-Response Relationships: Examine evidence from studies that have explored dose-response relationships between dietary factors and cancer risk, including optimal intake levels for specific nutrients or food groups.

12. Consensus Statements and Guidelines: Highlight consensus statements and guidelines from reputable organisations, such as the World Cancer Research Fund (WCRF) and the American Institute for Cancer Research (AICR), that synthesise evidence from scientific studies to provide recommendations for cancer prevention through diet and lifestyle.

Chapter 2: Stocking Your Anticancer Kitchen

Essential Anti-Cancer Foods

Exploring essential anti-cancer foods is crucial for understanding which dietary choices may help reduce cancer risk. Here's how to structure this topic.

1. Anti-Cancer Foods: Begin by emphasising the importance of incorporating nutrient-rich foods into the diet to support overall health and reduce the risk of cancer. Highlight that certain foods contain bioactive compounds with potential anti-cancer properties.

2. Fruits and Vegetables: Discuss the importance of consuming a variety of colourful fruits and vegetables, which are rich in vitamins, minerals, antioxidants, and phytochemicals. Highlight specific examples of anti-cancer fruits and vegetables, such as berries, leafy greens, cruciferous vegetables, citrus fruits, and tomatoes.

3. Whole Grains: Explore the benefits of whole grains, which are high in fibre, vitamins, minerals, and phytochemicals. Discuss how consuming whole grains, such as oats, brown rice, quinoa, and whole wheat, may help reduce the risk of colorectal cancer and other types of cancer.

4. Legumes: Examine the role of legumes, including beans, lentils, chickpeas, and peas, in cancer prevention. Discuss how legumes are rich in fibre, protein, vitamins, minerals, and phytochemicals, which may help lower the risk of various cancers, including colorectal cancer.

5. Healthy Fats: Discuss the importance of consuming healthy fats, such as those found in fatty fish, nuts, seeds, avocados, and olive oil. Highlight how omega-3 fatty acids and monounsaturated fats have anti-inflammatory properties and may help reduce the risk of certain cancers, such as breast and prostate cancer.

6. Herbs and Spices: Explore the potential anti-cancer properties of herbs and spices, which are rich in antioxidants and phytochemicals. Highlight specific examples, such as turmeric, ginger, garlic, cinnamon, and oregano, and discuss how they may help inhibit cancer cell growth and inflammation.

7. Teas: Examine the benefits of drinking tea, particularly green tea and black tea, which contain polyphenols and catechins with potential anti-cancer properties. Discuss how tea consumption may help reduce the risk of various cancers, including breast, prostate, and colorectal cancer.

8. Cruciferous Vegetables: Highlight the importance of consuming cruciferous vegetables, such as broccoli, cauliflower, Brussels sprouts, kale, and cabbage, which contain sulforaphane and other compounds with potential anti-cancer effects. Discuss how these vegetables may help inhibit cancer cell growth and promote detoxification.

9. Berries: Discuss the potential anti-cancer properties of berries, such as strawberries, blueberries, raspberries, and blackberries, which are rich in antioxidants, vitamins, and phytochemicals. Highlight how berry consumption may help reduce inflammation and oxidative stress, which are linked to cancer development.

10. Recommendations: Summarise key anti-cancer foods and their potential benefits for reducing cancer risk. Provide practical recommendations for incorporating these foods into a balanced diet to support overall health and well-being.

Organising Your Pantry

Organising your pantry is crucial for maintaining a healthy and efficient kitchen, especially when aiming to incorporate anti-cancer foods into your diet. Highlight the importance of a well-organised pantry for meal preparation, reducing food waste, and ensuring easy access to healthy ingredients.

1. Assessing Your Pantry: Begin by assessing your current pantry setup. Identify any expired or unhealthy items that need to be discarded and take inventory of staple ingredients that you use regularly.

2. Clearing Clutter: Discuss the importance of decluttering your pantry to create space for healthy foods. Remove any unnecessary items or duplicates to streamline your pantry storage.

3. Grouping Similar Items: Organise your pantry by grouping similar items together. Create designated sections for grains, beans, canned goods, spices, condiments, baking supplies, and snacks.

4. Storage Containers: Invest in airtight storage containers to keep ingredients fresh and organized. Transfer items like grains, nuts, seeds, and dried fruits into clear containers with labels for easy identification.

5. Labelling: Label storage containers and shelves to ensure everything has a designated place. Use a labelling system that is clear and easy to read, such as adhesive labels or chalkboard stickers.

6. Accessibility: Arrange your pantry so that frequently used items are easily accessible. Place everyday essentials at eye level or within arm's reach for convenience.

6. Maximising Space: Utilise vertical space by installing shelves or stacking bins to maximise storage capacity. Consider installing hooks or racks on the inside of pantry doors for additional storage options.

7. Rotation System: Implement a rotation system to ensure that older items are used first. Place newer purchases behind older ones to encourage FIFO (first in, first out) rotation.

8. Healthy Options Front and Center: Place healthy, anti-cancer foods like whole grains, legumes, nuts, seeds, and canned vegetables front and centre in your pantry to encourage their use in meal preparation.

9. Meal Prep Supplies: Dedicate a section of your pantry to meal prep supplies, such as reusable containers, meal prep bags, and portion control tools, to support healthy eating habits.

10. Emergency Kit: Create an emergency kit in your pantry stocked with non-perishable items like canned soups, beans, tuna, and shelf-stable grains for quick and easy meal options during busy times or emergencies.

11. Regular Maintenance: Establish a routine for pantry maintenance, such as weekly or monthly checks to ensure items are organised, labelled, and in good condition. Take the opportunity to restock essentials as needed.

12. Final Tips: Summarise key points for organising your pantry and maintaining a healthy kitchen environment. Encourage readers to customise their pantry organisation system to suit their needs and lifestyle.

Shopping Tips for Anti-Cancer Ingredients

When shopping for anti-cancer ingredients, it's important to make informed choices to ensure you're selecting the healthiest options available. Here's how to structure this topic.

1. Plan Ahead: Begin by planning your meals for the week and creating a shopping list based on anti-cancer foods you want to incorporate into your diet. This helps streamline the shopping process and prevents impulse purchases.

2. Choose Whole Foods: Opt for whole, minimally processed foods whenever possible. Focus on fresh fruits and vegetables, whole grains, legumes, lean proteins, nuts, seeds, and healthy fats.

3. Read Labels: Take time to read food labels and ingredient lists. Avoid products with added sugars, unhealthy fats (such as trans fats), artificial additives, and preservatives.

4. Prioritise Produce: Allocate a significant portion of your shopping trip to the produce section. Choose a variety of colourful fruits and vegetables, aiming to include a rainbow of colours to maximise nutrient intake.

5. Buy Organic When Possible: Consider purchasing organic produce, especially for items on the Environmental Working Group's "Dirty Dozen" list, which are known to contain higher levels of pesticide residues.

6. Select Seasonal Produce: Opt for seasonal fruits and vegetables, as they are often fresher, more flavorful, and may contain higher levels of nutrients compared to out-of-season produce.

7. Explore Farmers Markets: Visit local farmers markets to find fresh, locally grown produce. Not only does this support local farmers, but it also allows you to access a wider variety of seasonal and organic options.

8. Choose Lean Proteins: Select lean protein sources such as poultry, fish, tofu, tempeh, beans, and legumes. Limit consumption of processed meats and opt for grass-fed, pasture-raised, or organic options when possible.

9. Include Plant-Based Proteins: Incorporate plant-based protein sources like beans, lentils, quinoa, and nuts into your shopping list. These foods are rich in fibre, vitamins, minerals, and phytochemicals that support overall health.

10. Diversify Your Grains: Choose a variety of whole grains such as brown rice, quinoa, oats, barley, and whole wheat pasta. Experiment with lesser-known grains like farro, freekeh, and bulgur for added variety and nutrition.

11. Stock Up on Herbs and Spices: Add flavour to your meals with herbs and spices that have anti-inflammatory and antioxidant properties. Include staples like turmeric, ginger, garlic, cinnamon, and oregano in your shopping cart.

12. Minimise Processed Foods: Limit purchases of processed and packaged foods, which often contain unhealthy additives, preservatives, and excessive amounts of salt, sugar, and unhealthy fats.

Tools and Gadgets for a Healthy Kitchen

1. High-Quality Knives: Investing in a set of high-quality knives, including a chef's knife, paring knife, and serrated knife, is essential. Sharp, durable knives not only make chopping fruits, vegetables, and other ingredients easier but also safer by reducing the risk of slips and cuts. A well-maintained knife can drastically improve your cooking efficiency and precision.

2. Cutting Boards: Use separate cutting boards for fruits and vegetables, and for meats, to avoid cross-contamination, which is crucial for food safety. Opt for sturdy, non-slip boards that are easy to clean. Consider materials like bamboo or plastic, which are gentle on your knives and easy to sanitise.

3. Blender: A high-powered blender is a versatile tool for making smoothies, soups, sauces, and nut butters. It allows you to blend a variety of fruits, vegetables, and other healthy ingredients into smooth, nutrient-dense meals and beverages. Blenders can also help in making plant-based milks and purees, facilitating a plant-based diet.

4. Food Processor: A food processor is indispensable for chopping, slicing, shredding, and pureeing ingredients quickly. It can handle large quantities of produce, making it easier to prepare salads, dips, dressings, and other healthy recipes. Food processors save time and effort, especially when dealing with tough vegetables and nuts.

5. Spiralizer: A spiralizer enables you to create vegetable noodles from zucchini, carrots, and other vegetables, offering a healthy, low-carb alternative to pasta. This tool encourages the inclusion of more vegetables in your diet, promoting a plant-based nutrition approach that is beneficial for cancer prevention.

6. Steamer Basket: A steamer basket is a simple yet effective tool for cooking vegetables, fish, and grains while preserving their nutrients. Steaming is a gentle cooking method that maintains the integrity of vitamins and minerals, ensuring that your meals are as nutritious as possible.

7. Instant Pot or Pressure Cooker: An Instant Pot or pressure cooker is a versatile appliance that can make soups, stews, grains, and legumes quickly and efficiently. These tools use high pressure to cook food faster, preserving nutrients and enhancing flavours. They are ideal for preparing nutrient-rich meals in a time-efficient manner.

8. Slow Cooker: A slow cooker is perfect for preparing healthy, hearty meals with minimal effort. It's excellent for cooking beans, lentils, and tough cuts of meat to tender perfection. Slow cooking allows for the gradual melding of flavours and retention of nutrients, making it a great tool for nutrient-rich meals.

9. Mandoline Slicer: A mandoline slicer allows for quick and even slicing of fruits and vegetables, which can enhance the presentation and texture of your dishes. It makes it easier to prepare salads, chips, and garnishes, encouraging the inclusion of a variety of vegetables in your diet.

10. Non-Stick Cookware: High-quality non-stick pans and pots reduce the need for excessive oil and fats in cooking, promoting healthier meal preparation. Non-stick surfaces ensure that food doesn't stick, making cooking and cleaning easier and supporting low-fat cooking methods.

11. Herb Scissors: Herb scissors make chopping fresh herbs quick and effortless. Fresh herbs add flavor and nutritional benefits to your meals without extra calories or sodium. They are rich in antioxidants and phytochemicals, which contribute to overall health and cancer prevention.

12. Salad Spinner: A salad spinner is essential for washing and drying leafy greens and herbs, ensuring they are clean and crisp for salads and other dishes. Properly dried greens improve the texture of your salads and prevent dilution of dressings.

Chapter 3: Superfoods That Fight Cancer

The Power of Berries and Fruits

Fruits, especially berries, are powerhouses of essential nutrients and bioactive compounds that can contribute significantly to cancer prevention and overall health. Here are 14 detailed points exploring their benefits and how to incorporate them into your diet:

1. Rich in Antioxidants: Berries and fruits are loaded with antioxidants, such as vitamin C, vitamin E, and various phytochemicals like flavonoids and polyphenols. These antioxidants help neutralise free radicals, reducing oxidative stress and potentially lowering cancer risk.
Examples: Blueberries, strawberries, and oranges are particularly high in antioxidants.

2. High in Fibre: Dietary fibre from fruits aids in digestion, helps maintain a healthy weight, and supports regular bowel movements. High-fibre diets are linked to a lower risk of colorectal cancer.
Examples: Apples, pears, and raspberries are excellent sources of dietary fiber.

3. Anti-Inflammatory Properties: Many berries and fruits have anti-inflammatory properties due to their high content of bioactive compounds. Chronic inflammation is a known risk factor for various cancers.

Examples: Pineapples contain bromelain, and cherries are rich in anthocyanins, both of which have anti-inflammatory effects.

4. Boosting Immune System:
The vitamins and minerals in fruits, particularly vitamin C, support a strong immune system, enhancing the body's ability to fight off infections and potentially cancer cells.

Examples: Citrus fruits like oranges, lemons, and grapefruits are well-known immune boosters.

5. Phytochemical Benefits: Phytochemicals, such as quercetin, resveratrol, and ellagic acid, found in berries and fruits, have been studied for their anti-cancer properties, including inhibiting tumor growth and inducing cancer cell death.

Examples: Grapes contain resveratrol, while strawberries and raspberries are rich in ellagic acid.

6. Low Glycemic Index: Many berries have a low glycemic index, meaning they do not cause rapid spikes in blood sugar levels. Stable blood sugar

levels are important for reducing the risk of type 2 diabetes, which is a risk factor for certain cancers.
Examples: Blueberries and blackberries are examples of low-glycemic fruits.

7. Hydration and Detoxification: Fruits like watermelon and cucumbers have high water content, helping to keep the body hydrated and aiding in detoxification, which can support overall health and cancer prevention.
Examples: Watermelon, cucumbers, and cantaloupe.

8. Supporting Gut Health: The fibre and natural prebiotics in fruits support a healthy gut microbiome, which plays a crucial role in immune function and inflammation regulation.
Examples: Bananas contain prebiotic fibres that feed beneficial gut bacteria.

9. Vitamin-Rich: Fruits are excellent sources of essential vitamins, such as vitamin A, C, and K, which play roles in maintaining healthy cells and tissues.
Examples: Mangoes are high in vitamin A, while kiwis are rich in vitamin C and K.

10. Cancer-Fighting Compounds: Specific compounds in fruits have been found to have anti-cancer properties. For instance, the ellagic acid in strawberries and raspberries has been shown to slow the growth of certain tumors.

Examples: Pomegranates contain punicalagins and punicic acid, which have anti-cancer properties.

11. Convenience and Versatility: Fruits are convenient and versatile, making them easy to incorporate into any diet. They can be eaten fresh, frozen, dried, or juiced, and added to a variety of dishes.

Examples: Berries can be added to smoothies, oatmeal, salads, or enjoyed as a snack.

12. Promoting Healthy Skin: The antioxidants and vitamins in fruits promote healthy skin, which is a visible indicator of overall health. Healthy skin reflects the internal health and can signify lower levels of inflammation.

Examples: Avocados are rich in healthy fats and vitamin E, both of which support skin health.

Cruciferous Vegetables, A Potent Ally

Cruciferous vegetables are among the most powerful foods when it comes to cancer prevention and overall health. They are packed with nutrients, bioactive compounds, and offer a wide range of health benefits. Here are detailed points explaining why cruciferous vegetables are a potent ally in the fight against cancer.

1. **Rich in Glucosinolates:** Cruciferous vegetables are rich in glucosinolates, sulfur-containing compounds that, when broken down during chewing and digestion, form biologically active compounds like isothiocyanates and indoles. These compounds have been shown to inhibit the development and growth of cancer cells.
Examples: Broccoli, Brussels sprouts, and kale are particularly high in glucosinolates.

2. **Detoxification Support:** The compounds in cruciferous vegetables enhance the body's detoxification systems. They promote the elimination of potential carcinogens by boosting the activity of detoxifying enzymes in the liver.
Examples: Cauliflower and cabbage support liver function and detoxification processes.

3. **Anti-Inflammatory Properties:** Chronic inflammation is a known risk factor for many types of cancer. Cruciferous vegetables contain anti-inflammatory compounds that can help reduce inflammation in the body, lowering cancer risk.
Examples: Arugula and radishes have anti-inflammatory properties.

4. Rich in Antioxidants: These vegetables are rich in antioxidants like vitamins C, E, and beta-carotene, which help protect cells from oxidative damage caused by free radicals. This can prevent the mutation of cells that could lead to cancer.
Examples: Turnips and collard greens are high in antioxidants.

5. High in Fiber: Dietary fiber from cruciferous vegetables aids digestion, promotes regular bowel movements, and can help lower the risk of colorectal cancer by keeping the digestive system healthy.
Examples: Broccoli and Brussels sprouts are excellent sources of dietary fibre.

6. Hormonal Balance: Certain compounds in cruciferous vegetables, like indole-3-carbinol, can help balance oestrogen levels in the body, which may reduce the risk of hormone-related cancers such as breast and prostate cancer.
Examples: Kale and bok choy contain indole-3-carbinol.

7. Immune System Boost: The vitamins, minerals, and bioactive compounds in cruciferous vegetables support a healthy immune system, enhancing the body's ability to fight off infections and abnormal cell growth.

Examples: Cabbage and watercress support immune function.

8. **Low-Calorie, Nutrient-Dense:** These vegetables are low in calories but high in essential nutrients, making them an excellent choice for maintaining a healthy weight and reducing obesity-related cancer risks.
Examples: Arugula and radishes are low in calories yet nutrient-rich.

9. **Sulforaphane Benefits:** Sulforaphane, a compound found in many cruciferous vegetables, has been shown to have strong anti-cancer properties by inhibiting histone deacetylase, an enzyme involved in cancer cell growth.
Examples: Broccoli sprouts are exceptionally high in sulforaphane.

10. **Support for Gut Health:** The fiber and prebiotic content of cruciferous vegetables support a healthy gut microbiome, which plays a crucial role in immune function and cancer prevention.
Examples: Cauliflower and cabbage are beneficial for gut health.

11. **Variety and Versatility:** Cruciferous vegetables come in many varieties and can be prepared in

numerous ways, making it easy to include them in your diet regularly.

Examples: Raw in salads, steamed, roasted, or stir-fried; try incorporating different cooking methods.

12. **Nutrient-Rich:** These vegetables are rich in essential vitamins (A, C, K) and minerals (folate, potassium, calcium) that are vital for maintaining overall health and supporting bodily functions.
Examples: Kale is rich in vitamins A, C, and K.

Whole Grains and Legumes

Whole grains and legumes are essential components of a healthy, anti-cancer diet. Let's take a closer look at their benefits.

Whole Grains:
1. Whole grains are rich in dietary fibre, which helps regulate digestion, prevents constipation, and reduces the risk of colon cancer by promoting the elimination of waste and toxins from the body.
2. The high fibre content in whole grains contributes to satiety, helping individuals feel fuller for longer periods. This can prevent overeating and aid in maintaining a healthy weight, reducing the risk of obesity-related cancers.
3. Whole grains have a low glycemic index, meaning they release glucose into the bloodstream slowly and

steadily. This helps prevent insulin resistance, a condition associated with an increased risk of developing certain types of cancer.

4. Whole grains contain essential B vitamins, including folate, which plays a crucial role in DNA synthesis and cell division. Inadequate folate intake has been linked to an increased risk of cancer, particularly in the colon and breast.

5. Whole grains are rich in minerals like iron, magnesium, and selenium. Iron supports the production of red blood cells and immune function, while magnesium and selenium are involved in various enzymatic reactions that promote overall health.

6. These grains contain a variety of phytonutrients, including phenols and flavonoids, which exhibit antioxidant and anti-inflammatory properties that can protect against cancer development.

7. Whole grains provide sustained energy due to their complex carbohydrate content, helping to maintain stable blood sugar levels and prevent unhealthy snacking between meals.

Legumes:

1. Legumes are packed with fibre, protein, and complex carbohydrates, providing sustained energy, promoting satiety, and helping maintain a healthy weight.

2. As an excellent source of plant-based protein, legumes support muscle mass maintenance and immune system function, both of which are crucial in cancer prevention.
3. Legumes are rich in essential vitamins and minerals, including folate, iron, magnesium, and potassium. These nutrients play vital roles in various bodily functions, including energy production, immune system support, and maintaining stable blood pressure.
4. Legumes contain various antioxidants and phytochemicals, such as flavonoids, saponins, and phytic acid, which have been shown to exhibit anti-cancer properties by neutralising free radicals and inhibiting cancer cell growth.
5. Similar to whole grains, legumes have a low glycemic index, which aids in blood sugar regulation and reduces inflammation a contributing factor to cancer development.
6. Legumes contain resistant starch, a type of carbohydrate that acts as a prebiotic, supporting gut health and potentially reducing the risk of colon cancer.
7. As nutrient-dense, low-fat food options, legumes are a heart-healthy choice for individuals concerned about reducing their cancer risk through diet.

Spices and Herbs with Anti-Cancer Properties

Spices and herbs are not just for flavor; they also offer significant health benefits, including anti-cancer properties. Here are detailed points explaining the roles of various spices and herbs in cancer prevention.

1. Turmeric (Curcumin): Turmeric contains curcumin, a compound with powerful anti-inflammatory and antioxidant effects. Curcumin has been shown to inhibit the growth of cancer cells and reduce the spread of tumours.
How to Use: Add turmeric to curries, soups, and smoothies, or take as a supplement.

2. Ginger: Ginger contains gingerol, which has anti-inflammatory and antioxidant properties. It can help reduce oxidative stress and inflammation, both of which are linked to cancer development.
How to Use: Incorporate fresh ginger into teas, stir-fries, and baked goods.

3. Garlic: Garlic is rich in sulphur compounds, such as allicin, which have been shown to enhance the immune system and reduce the risk of certain cancers, including stomach and colorectal cancers.

How to Use: Use fresh garlic in sauces, dressings, and roasted vegetables.

4. Cinnamon: Cinnamon contains cinnamaldehyde, which has antioxidant properties and can inhibit the growth of cancer cells. It also helps regulate blood sugar levels, reducing cancer risk factors like obesity.
How to Use: Sprinkle cinnamon on oatmeal, yogurt, and in baking recipes.

5. Oregano: Oregano is high in antioxidants and contains compounds like carvacrol and thymol, which have anti-cancer properties. Oregano can help reduce oxidative stress and inflammation.
How to Use: Add dried or fresh oregano to pasta sauces, salads, and marinades.

6. Rosemary: Rosemary contains carnosol and rosmarinic acid, both of which have been shown to inhibit the growth of cancer cells and reduce inflammation.
How to Use: Use rosemary in roasted meats, vegetables, and infused oils.

7. Thyme: Thyme contains thymol, which has strong antioxidant properties and can help protect cells from damage that may lead to cancer.

How to Use: Incorporate thyme in soups, stews, and roasted dishes.

8. Basil: Basil is rich in antioxidants, including eugenol, which can help fight inflammation and reduce the risk of cancer. Basil also boosts the immune system.
How to Use: Use fresh basil in pesto, salads, and as a garnish for various dishes.

9. Parsley: Parsley contains apigenin, a compound that has been shown to have anti-cancer effects, particularly in breast and colon cancers. It helps inhibit the growth of cancer cells.
How to Use: Add fresh parsley to salads, soups, and smoothies.

10. Mint: Mint contains menthol, which has anti-inflammatory and antioxidant properties. It can help reduce oxidative stress and improve digestion, which is linked to cancer prevention.
How to Use: Use fresh mint in teas, salads, and desserts.

11. Cayenne Pepper (Capsaicin): Cayenne pepper contains capsaicin, which has been shown to inhibit the growth of cancer cells and induce apoptosis (programmed cell death) in various cancer types.

How to Use: Add cayenne pepper to spicy dishes, soups, and sauces.

12. Sage: Sage is rich in antioxidants like rosmarinic acid and carnosic acid, which can help protect cells from DNA damage and reduce the risk of cancer.
How to Use: Use sage in stuffing, soups, and meat dishes.

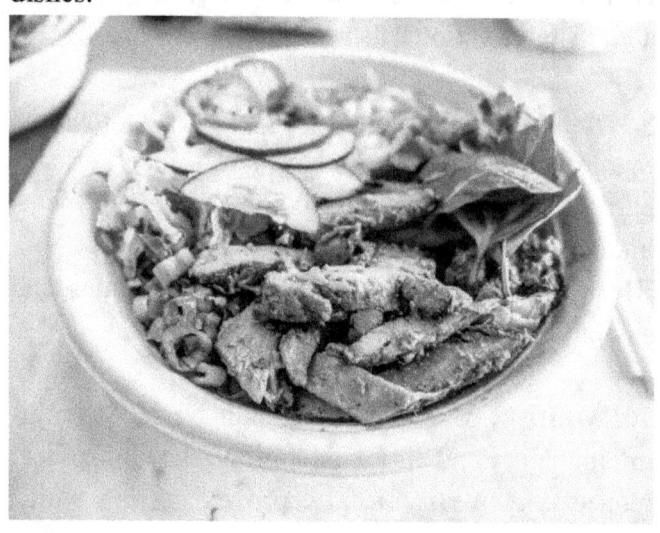

Chapter 4: Anti-Cancer Breakfasts

Energising Smoothies

Energising smoothies are a delicious and convenient way to pack essential nutrients into your diet, supporting overall health and providing specific anti-cancer benefits. Here are detailed points explaining how to create and enjoy smoothies that help fight cancer.

1. Green Smoothie with Spinach and Kale: Spinach and kale are rich in antioxidants and anti-cancer compounds such as sulforaphane and indole-3-carbinol. These leafy greens support detoxification and reduce inflammation.
Recipe Idea: Blend spinach, kale, a banana, and almond milk for a nutrient-packed green smoothie.

2. Berry Antioxidant Blast: Berries, including blueberries, strawberries, and raspberries, are high in vitamins, fibre, and antioxidants like ellagic acid and anthocyanins, which help protect cells from damage.
Recipe Idea: Combine mixed berries, Greek yoghourt, and a splash of orange juice for a refreshing smoothie.

3. Turmeric Mango Smoothie: Turmeric's active compound, curcumin, has powerful anti-inflammatory and anti-cancer properties. Mango adds a sweet flavour and is rich in vitamins A and C.
Recipe Idea: Blend mango chunks, a teaspoon of turmeric, a pinch of black pepper, and coconut milk for a vibrant smoothie.

4. Beet and Berry Detox Smoothie: Beets contain betalains, which have antioxidant and anti-inflammatory properties. Paired with berries, this smoothie supports liver detoxification and overall health.
Recipe Idea: Blend cooked beets, mixed berries, a splash of lemon juice, and water for a detoxifying drink.

5. Almond and Oat Smoothie: Almonds provide healthy fats and vitamin E, while oats add fiber and help maintain stable blood sugar levels. This combination supports heart health and energy.
Recipe Idea: Combine soaked oats, almond butter, a banana, and unsweetened almond milk for a creamy, filling smoothie.

6. Pineapple and Spinach Smoothie: Pineapple is rich in bromelain, an enzyme with anti-inflammatory properties, and spinach adds a dose of iron and antioxidants.

Recipe Idea: Blend pineapple chunks, fresh spinach, a banana, and coconut water for a tropical, nutrient-dense smoothie.

7. Chia Seed Superfood Smoothie: Chia seeds are high in omega-3 fatty acids, fibre, and antioxidants, which support heart health and reduce inflammation.
Recipe Idea: Mix chia seeds, blueberries, a banana, and unsweetened almond milk for a smoothie packed with superfoods.

8. Carrot and Apple Smoothie: Carrots are high in beta-carotene, which converts to vitamin A in the body and has antioxidant properties. Apples add fibre and vitamin C.
Recipe Idea: Blend carrots, an apple, a small piece of ginger, and orange juice for a sweet, nutritious smoothie.

9. Protein-Packed Smoothie: Adding a protein source like Greek yoghourt or plant-based protein powder helps repair and build tissues and maintain muscle mass, which is crucial during cancer recovery.
Recipe Idea: Combine Greek yogurt, mixed berries, a scoop of protein powder, and water for a protein-rich smoothie.

10. Avocado and Berry Smoothie: Avocados are rich in healthy fats and antioxidants like lutein, which support overall health and help reduce inflammation.
Recipe Idea: Blend half an avocado, mixed berries, a banana, and almond milk for a creamy, nutrient-dense smoothie.

11. Cucumber and Mint Smoothie: Cucumbers are hydrating and contain antioxidants, while mint adds a refreshing flavour and aids digestion.
Recipe Idea: Mix cucumber, fresh mint leaves, a lime, and coconut water for a hydrating, refreshing smoothie.

12. Flaxseed and Banana Smoothie: Flaxseeds are high in lignans and omega-3 fatty acids, which have been shown to have anti-cancer properties and support heart health.
Recipe Idea: Blend a tablespoon of flaxseeds, a banana, spinach, and unsweetened almond milk for a heart-healthy smoothie.

Nutrient-Packed Oatmeals

Oatmeals are a versatile and nutritious breakfast option that can be tailored to include a variety of cancer-fighting ingredients. Here are points explaining how to create and enjoy nutrient-packed oatmeals that help in cancer prevention and overall health.

1. Berry Blast Oatmeal: Berries are high in antioxidants, fiber, and vitamins, which help protect cells from damage and reduce cancer risk.
Recipe Idea: Top cooked oats with a mix of fresh blueberries, strawberries, and raspberries. Add a drizzle of honey and a sprinkle of chia seeds.

2. Turmeric Golden Oatmeal: Turmeric contains curcumin, a compound with potent anti-inflammatory and anti-cancer properties.
Recipe Idea: Stir a teaspoon of turmeric and a pinch of black pepper into your oatmeal. Add almond milk, a banana, and a sprinkle of cinnamon for flavor.

3. Apple Cinnamon Oatmeal: Apples are rich in fiber and vitamin C, while cinnamon has anti-inflammatory and antioxidant properties.
Recipe Idea: Cook oats with diced apples, a teaspoon of cinnamon, and a handful of raisins. Top with chopped walnuts for added crunch and omega-3 fatty acids.

4. Green Smoothie Oatmeal: Spinach and kale are packed with vitamins, minerals, and cancer-fighting antioxidants.

Recipe Idea: Blend a handful of spinach or kale with a banana and almond milk. Pour the smoothie over cooked oats and top with fresh berries and chia seeds.

5. Ginger Peach Oatmeal: Ginger has anti-inflammatory properties, and peaches are high in vitamins A and C.
Recipe Idea: Cook oats with diced peaches and grated fresh ginger. Sweeten with a bit of honey and top with sliced almonds.

6. Pumpkin Spice Oatmeal: Pumpkin is rich in beta-carotene, fibre, and antioxidants that support immune health and reduce cancer risk.
Recipe Idea: Stir pumpkin puree, a teaspoon of cinnamon, and a pinch of nutmeg into your oatmeal. Top with a dollop of Greek yoghourt and a sprinkle of pumpkin seeds.

7. Blueberry Almond Oatmeal: Blueberries are rich in antioxidants, and almonds provide vitamin E and healthy fats.
Recipe Idea: Cook oats with fresh or frozen blueberries and top with sliced almonds and a drizzle of maple syrup.

8. Carrot Cake Oatmeal: Carrots are high in beta-carotene, and spices like cinnamon and nutmeg add antioxidants.
Recipe Idea: Stir grated carrots, a teaspoon of cinnamon, and a pinch of nutmeg into your oatmeal. Top with chopped walnuts and a spoonful of Greek yoghourt.

9. Chia Seed and Berry Oatmeal: Chia seeds are high in omega-3 fatty acids, fibre, and antioxidants, which support heart health and reduce inflammation.
Recipe Idea: Add a tablespoon of chia seeds to your cooked oats and top with fresh berries and a drizzle of honey.

10. Coconut and Mango Oatmeal: Coconut provides healthy fats, and mango is rich in vitamins A and C, which boost the immune system.
Recipe Idea: Stir coconut milk and diced mango into your oatmeal. Top with shredded coconut and a sprinkle of chia seeds.

11. Chocolate Avocado Oatmeal: Avocado provides healthy fats and antioxidants, while dark chocolate contains flavonoids that can reduce cancer risk.
Recipe Idea: Mash half an avocado into your cooked oats and stir in a tablespoon of unsweetened cocoa

powder. Top with a few dark chocolate chips and sliced almonds.

12. Flaxseed and Berry Oatmeal: Flaxseeds are rich in lignans and omega-3 fatty acids, which have anti-cancer properties.
Recipe Idea: Stir a tablespoon of ground flaxseeds into your cooked oats and top with a mix of fresh berries and a splash of almond milk.

Anti-Cancer Breakfast Bowls

A great way to start your day is with a nutrient-packed anti-cancer breakfast bowl. These bowls combine a variety of healing foods to provide a powerful dose of nutrients that can help prevent cancer. Let's delve into how to create these bowls and why they are beneficial.

1. Fruits, Antioxidant-Rich Berries: Top your bowl with a variety of berries such as blueberries, strawberries, and raspberries. These fruits are known for their high antioxidant content.
Benefits: Antioxidants neutralise free radicals in the body, reducing oxidative stress and potentially lowering the risk of cancer. Berries are also rich in vitamins C and K and fibre.

2. Proteins, Nuts and Seeds: Add nuts and seeds like almonds, chia seeds, flaxseeds, or walnuts to your breakfast bowl. These ingredients provide a good source of plant-based protein and healthy fats.
Benefits: Nuts and seeds contain omega-3 fatty acids, which have anti-inflammatory properties and may reduce the risk of cancer. They also provide protein for muscle repair and growth, and help keep you full longer.

3. Vegetables, Leafy Greens and Cruciferous Veggies: Include a handful of leafy greens such as spinach, kale, or arugula, and cruciferous vegetables like broccoli sprouts.
Benefits: Leafy greens are packed with vitamins, minerals, and antioxidants. Cruciferous vegetables contain sulforaphane, a compound with potent anti-cancer properties. These vegetables help detoxify the body and support overall health.

4. Healthy Fats, Avocado and Coconut: Incorporate slices of avocado or a sprinkle of unsweetened coconut flakes. These ingredients provide healthy fats essential for brain function and overall health.
Benefits: Healthy fats support cell structure and function. Avocados are rich in monounsaturated fats, which are heart-healthy, while coconut contains

medium-chain triglycerides (MCTs) that provide quick energy.

5. Probiotics, Yogurt or Kefir: Add a dollop of plain yoghourt or kefir to your bowl. These fermented foods are rich in probiotics.
Benefits: Probiotics promote a healthy gut microbiome, which is essential for immune function and overall health. A balanced gut flora can help reduce inflammation and potentially lower cancer risk.

6. Whole Grains for Fibre: Use quinoa, oats, or brown rice to ensure a high fibre intake.

7. Antioxidant-Rich Berries: Include blueberries, strawberries, and raspberries to fight free radicals.

8. Plant-Based Proteins: Add nuts and seeds like almonds and chia seeds for protein and healthy fats.
9. Leafy Greens: Incorporate spinach or kale for a boost of vitamins and minerals.

10. Cruciferous Vegetables: Use broccoli sprouts to benefit from sulforaphane.

Healthy Morning Beverages

Starting your day with a nutritious beverage sets the tone for healthy choices throughout the day. Here are some options for morning beverages that not only taste delicious but also provide essential nutrients to support your anti-cancer journey.

1. Green Tea: Green tea is rich in antioxidants called catechins, which have been linked to reduced cancer risk. It helps boost metabolism, aids in weight management, and supports overall health.

2. Turmeric Latte: A warming blend of turmeric, milk (or plant-based milk), and spices like cinnamon and ginger. Turmeric contains curcumin, a compound with potent anti-inflammatory and antioxidant properties.

3. Berry Blast Smoothie: A refreshing blend of mixed berries, spinach or kale, banana, and a splash of almond milk or yoghurt. Berries are packed with antioxidants and vitamins, while leafy greens provide fibre and essential nutrients.

4. Golden Milk: A traditional Ayurvedic beverage made with turmeric, milk (or plant-based milk), black pepper, and honey. Turmeric and black pepper work synergistically to enhance the bioavailability of curcumin, maximising its anti-inflammatory effects.

5. Matcha Latte: Matcha is a powdered form of green tea, whisked with hot water or milk (or plant-based milk). It contains higher concentrations of antioxidants compared to regular green tea, providing a sustained energy boost without the crash.

6. Ginger Lemon Detox Drink: A revitalising combination of fresh ginger, lemon juice, and water, optionally sweetened with honey. Ginger aids digestion, supports immune function, and has anti-inflammatory properties, while lemon provides vitamin C and promotes detoxification.

7. Probiotic Smoothie: A creamy blend of kefir or yoghurt, mixed with fruits like banana, mango, or pineapple. Probiotics in kefir or yoghurt support gut health, which is linked to overall immunity and cancer prevention.

8. Warm Lemon Water: A simple yet effective beverage made by squeezing fresh lemon juice into warm water. Lemon water alkalizes the body, aids digestion, and provides a dose of vitamin C to support immune function.

9. Carrot Juice: A vibrant and nutritious juice made from fresh carrots, ginger, and orange, optionally combined with other vegetables like spinach, kale, or beets. Carrots are rich in beta-carotene and other antioxidants, which support immune function and help reduce inflammation.

10. **Apple Cider Vinegar Drink:** A tangy and refreshing tonic made with a tablespoon of raw, unfiltered apple cider vinegar diluted in water, sweetened with honey or stevia. Apple cider vinegar aids digestion, supports weight management, and has been linked to a reduced risk of certain cancers.

11. **Herbal Infusions:** Various herbal teas, such as chamomile, peppermint, or rooibos, provide calming and soothing effects while offering antioxidants and other health-boosting compounds.

12. **Water with Cucumber and Mint:** A hydrating and refreshing drink made by infusing water with sliced cucumber and fresh mint leaves. Cucumber provides hydration and essential nutrients, while mint aids digestion and adds a refreshing flavour.

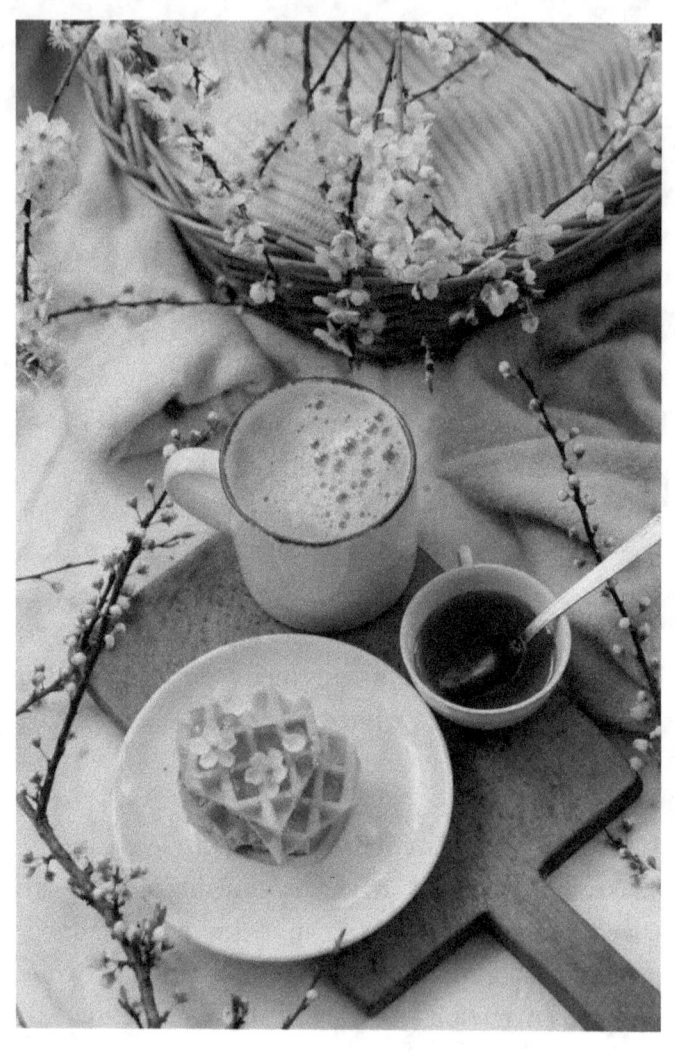

Chapter 5: Immune-Boosting Lunches

Superfood Salads

Superfood salads are a delicious and nutritious way to incorporate a variety of nutrient-dense ingredients into your diet. Here's how to create vibrant salads packed with anti-cancer nutrients.

1. Leafy Greens Base: Start with a base of leafy greens such as kale, spinach, or arugula. These greens are rich in vitamins, minerals, and antioxidants.
Benefits: Leafy greens contain compounds like sulforaphane and chlorophyll, which have been shown to have anti-cancer properties and support overall health.

2. Colourful Vegetables: Add a variety of colourful vegetables like bell peppers, carrots, cucumbers, and cherry tomatoes. These vegetables provide a range of vitamins, minerals, and phytochemicals.
Benefits: The vibrant colours of vegetables indicate the presence of antioxidants such as beta-carotene, vitamin C, and lycopene, which help protect cells from damage and reduce cancer risk.

3. Protein Power: Incorporate plant-based proteins like beans, lentils, chickpeas, or tofu. These proteins are rich in fibre and essential amino acids.

Benefits: Plant-based proteins help maintain a healthy weight, support muscle growth and repair, and reduce the risk of chronic diseases, including cancer.

4. Healthy Fats: Include sources of healthy fats such as avocado, nuts, seeds, or olives. These fats provide satiety and support brain health.

Benefits: Healthy fats contain omega-3 fatty acids, which have anti-inflammatory properties and may reduce the risk of cancer development and progression.

5. Berries and Citrus: Add antioxidant-rich fruits like berries (strawberries, blueberries, raspberries) and citrus fruits (orange segments, grapefruit slices).

Benefits: Berries and citrus fruits are packed with vitamin C and other antioxidants that help neutralise free radicals, reduce inflammation, and support immune function.

6. Powerhouse Herbs: Incorporate fresh herbs like parsley, cilantro, basil, or mint for flavor and additional nutrients.

Benefits: Herbs contain unique phytonutrients and antioxidants that support detoxification, reduce inflammation, and enhance the flavour of salads.

7. Homemade Dressing: Make your own salad dressing using healthy fats like olive oil, vinegar or citrus juice, and herbs/spices.
Benefits: Homemade dressings allow you to control the ingredients and avoid added sugars, unhealthy fats, and artificial additives often found in store-bought dressings.

8. Leafy Greens Base: Kale, spinach, or arugula provide essential nutrients and antioxidants.

9. Colourful Vegetables: Bell peppers, carrots, cucumbers, and cherry tomatoes offer a variety of vitamins and minerals.

10. Protein Power: Beans, lentils, chickpeas, or tofu provide plant-based protein and fibre.

11. Healthy Fats: Avocado, nuts, seeds, or olives contribute omega-3 fatty acids and satiety.

12. Berries and Citrus: Strawberries, blueberries, raspberries, oranges, or grapefruits add antioxidants and vitamin C.

Nutritious Grain Bowls

Nutritious grain bowls are versatile, satisfying, and packed with essential nutrients. Here's how to create hearty grain bowls that support your anti-cancer journey.

1. Leafy Greens: Add a generous serving of leafy greens like spinach, kale, or Swiss chard. These greens are loaded with antioxidants and phytonutrients.
Benefits: Leafy greens support detoxification, provide essential vitamins and minerals, and have anti-inflammatory properties.

2. Colourful Vegetables: Incorporate a variety of colourful vegetables such as bell peppers, broccoli, carrots, and cherry tomatoes. These vegetables provide a range of antioxidants and micronutrients.
Benefits: Colourful vegetables contain phytochemicals that help protect cells from damage, support immune function, and reduce cancer risk.

3. Lean Protein: Include lean protein sources like grilled chicken, tofu, tempeh, or beans. These proteins are essential for muscle repair and immune function.
Benefits: Lean proteins provide amino acids necessary for cellular repair, support a healthy metabolism, and help maintain muscle mass.

4. Healthy Fats: Add sources of healthy fats such as avocado, nuts, seeds, or olive oil. These fats provide satiety and support brain health.
Benefits: Healthy fats contain omega-3 fatty acids, which have anti-inflammatory properties and may help reduce the risk of cancer progression.

5. Flavorful Dressing or Sauce: Drizzle your grain bowl with a flavorful dressing or sauce made from ingredients like olive oil, lemon juice, herbs, and spices.
Benefits: A delicious dressing enhances the taste of your bowl and encourages consumption of nutrient-rich ingredients.

6. Optional Toppings: Add optional toppings such as crumbled feta cheese, dried fruit, roasted nuts, or seeds for extra flavour and texture.
Benefits: Toppings provide additional nutrients, texture, and flavour, making your grain bowl more satisfying and enjoyable.

7. Colourful Vegetables: Bell peppers, broccoli, carrots, and cherry tomatoes provide a variety of antioxidants and micronutrients.

8. Lean Protein: Grilled chicken, tofu, tempeh, or beans supply essential amino acids for cellular repair.

9. Healthy Fats: Avocado, nuts, seeds, or olive oil contribute omega-3 fatty acids and satiety.

10. Flavorful Dressing or Sauce: Olive oil, lemon juice, herbs, and spices create a delicious dressing to enhance the taste of your bowl.

Hearty Soups and Stews

Soups and stews are comforting dishes that can be both nourishing and beneficial in promoting an anti-cancer lifestyle. Here are some delicious and nutritious soup and stew ideas to incorporate into your meal plan1.

1. Nutritious Base: Using vegetable or bone broth as the base of your soup or stew not only adds flavour but also provides essential nutrients like vitamins and minerals. Homemade broths can be made with a variety of vegetables and herbs, enhancing both taste and nutritional value.

2. Abundance of Vegetables: Loading your soup or stew with colourful vegetables ensures you're getting a wide range of vitamins, minerals, and antioxidants. Carrots, celery, onions, and leafy greens are excellent choices, adding both flavour and nutrition.

3. Whole Grains or Legumes: Adding whole grains like barley, quinoa, or brown rice, as well as legumes such as lentils or chickpeas, boosts the fibre and protein content of your dish. These ingredients also contribute to a feeling of fullness and satisfaction.

4. Lean Protein: Incorporating lean protein sources like chicken breast, turkey, or tofu adds satiety and supports muscle repair and growth. Opting for lean cuts of meat or plant-based proteins keeps your dish light and nutritious.

5. Herbs and Spices: Seasoning your soup or stew with herbs and spices not only enhances the flavour but also provides additional health benefits. Garlic, ginger, turmeric, and thyme are known for their anti-inflammatory and antioxidant properties.

6. Healthy Fats: Adding a source of healthy fats like olive oil or avocado at the end of cooking adds richness and depth to your soup or stew. These fats are essential for nutrient absorption and provide a feeling of satisfaction.

7. Variety of Textures: Including ingredients with different textures, such as potatoes for creaminess or beans for bite, adds interest to your dish and keeps it visually appealing.

8. Low Sodium Options: Opting for low-sodium broths or making your own allows you to control the salt content of your soup or stew. Excessive sodium intake is linked to high blood pressure and other health issues, so it's important to monitor your intake.

9. Cooking Techniques: Slow cooking or pressure cooking soups and stews allows flavours to meld together and ingredients to become tender. These cooking methods result in a rich, flavorful dish with minimal effort.

10. Balanced Macronutrients: Aim to include a balance of carbohydrates, protein, and healthy fats in your soup or stew to create a well-rounded meal that keeps you satisfied and energised.

12. Portion Control: Pay attention to portion sizes when serving your soup or stew to avoid overeating. While these dishes are nutritious, consuming too much can lead to excess calorie intake.

Anti-Cancer Sandwiches and Wraps

1. Wholesome Ingredients: Selecting fresh vegetables, lean proteins, and whole grains ensures that your sandwiches and wraps are packed with essential nutrients, including vitamins, minerals, and fibre, which are crucial for overall health and wellbeing.

2. Fiber-Rich: Whole grain bread and wraps are rich in dietary fibre, which promotes healthy digestion, helps maintain a healthy weight, and may lower the risk of certain cancers, such as colorectal cancer.

3. Lean Proteins: Choosing lean protein sources such as grilled chicken, turkey, or tofu provides essential amino acids necessary for cell repair and maintenance, without the saturated fat content found in processed meats, which has been linked to an increased risk of cancer.

4. Healthy Fats: Adding sources of healthy fats like avocado, hummus, or olive oil not only enhances the flavour and texture of your sandwiches and wraps but also provides omega-3 fatty acids and monounsaturated fats, which have anti-inflammatory properties and may help reduce the risk of cancer.

5. Herbs and Spices: Incorporating herbs and spices like basil, cilantro, and turmeric not only adds flavour but also provides additional health benefits, as many herbs and spices contain potent antioxidants and anti-inflammatory compounds that may help protect against cancer.

6. Customizable Options: By allowing for customization, individuals can tailor their sandwiches and wraps to their taste preferences and dietary needs, ensuring that they enjoy their meals while still reaping the health benefits of the ingredients.

7. Portion Control: Paying attention to portion sizes helps prevent overeating, promotes weight management, and ensures that you're consuming a balanced meal with the right amount of nutrients.

8. Low Sodium: Choosing low-sodium condiments and ingredients helps reduce sodium intake, which is important for maintaining healthy blood pressure levels and reducing the risk of cardiovascular disease, a common comorbidity of cancer.

9. Quick and Easy: These recipes are designed to be simple and convenient, making them suitable for individuals with busy lifestyles who may not have the time for elaborate meal preparation.

10. Meal Prep Friendly: Preparing ingredients ahead of time makes it easier to assemble sandwiches and wraps quickly, whether you're packing lunch for work or school, saving time and ensuring that healthy options are readily available.

11. Kid-Friendly Options: Creating kid-friendly sandwich and wrap ideas encourages children to enjoy healthy foods from a young age, fostering lifelong habits that support overall health and well-being.

12. Allergen Alternatives be: Offering allergen-friendly options ensures that individuals with dietary restrictions can still enjoy delicious and nutritious sandwiches and wraps, promoting inclusivity and accessibility.

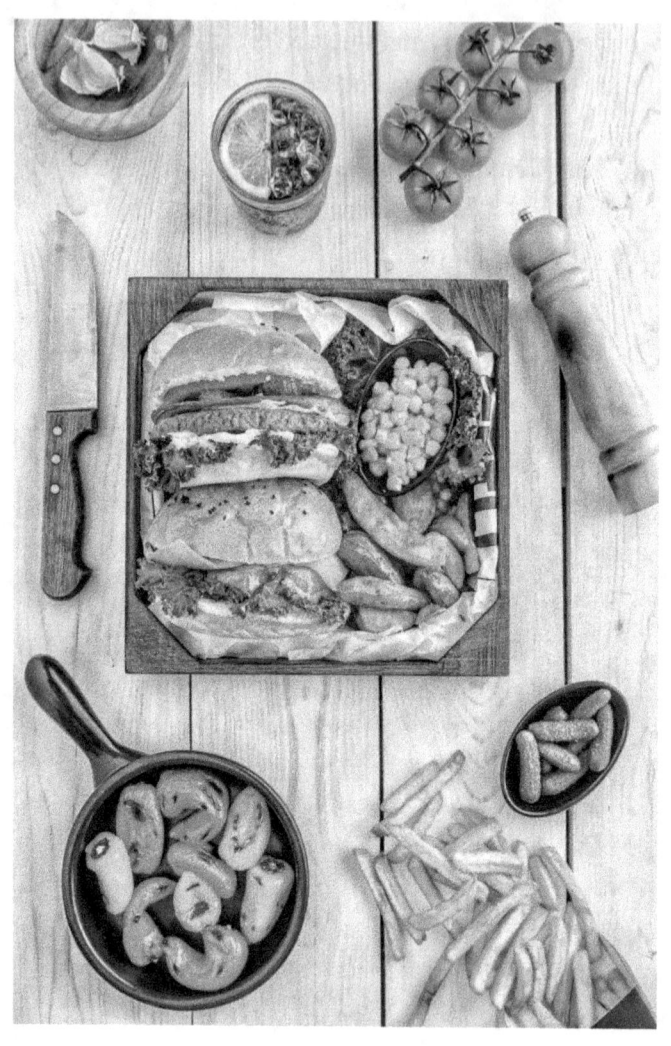

Chapter 6: Delicious and Healthy Dinners

Plant-Based Main Courses

In this chapter, we embark on a culinary journey celebrating the versatility and nourishment of plant-based cuisine. Plant-based main courses not only offer a spectrum of flavours and textures but also serve as a cornerstone of a cancer-fighting diet. From hearty legume-based stews to vibrant vegetable stir-fries, each recipe showcases the abundance of plant-derived nutrients that promote optimal health and resilience. Whether you're a committed vegan or simply looking to incorporate more plant-powered meals into your diet, these plant-based main courses provide a delicious and satisfying way to support your body's natural defences against cancer and other chronic diseases.

1. Nutrient Density: Plant-based main courses are rich in essential vitamins, minerals, and phytonutrients, providing a diverse array of nutrients crucial for maintaining overall health and vitality.

2. Fibre-Rich: Plant-based meals are naturally high in dietary fibre, which supports digestive health, promotes satiety, and may lower the risk of colorectal cancer.

3. Antioxidant Powerhouse: Fruits, vegetables, legumes, nuts, and seeds found in plant-based dishes are packed with antioxidants that help neutralise harmful free radicals, reducing oxidative stress and inflammation in the body.

4. Heart Health: Plant-based diets are associated with a lower risk of heart disease, a common comorbidity of cancer, due to their cholesterol-lowering, blood pressure-regulating, and anti-inflammatory properties.

5. Cancer-Fighting Phytochemicals: Phytochemicals found in plant foods, such as flavonoids, carotenoids, and polyphenols, have been shown to inhibit cancer cell growth, promote apoptosis (cell death), and suppress angiogenesis (the formation of new blood vessels to tumours).

6. Protein Richnes: Contrary to common misconceptions, plant-based diets can provide an ample amount of protein through sources like beans, lentils, tofu, tempeh, quinoa, and nuts, supporting muscle maintenance, repair, and overall body function.

7. Low in Saturated Fat: Plant-based main courses are naturally low in saturated fat and cholesterol, contributing to better cardiovascular health and reducing the risk of obesity-related cancers.

8. Environmental Sustainability: Choosing plant-based meals over animal products helps reduce greenhouse gas emissions, conserve water and land resources, and mitigate environmental degradation, promoting a more sustainable food system.

9. Ethical Considerations: Many individuals adopt plant-based diets for ethical reasons, including concerns about animal welfare and the environmental impact of animal agriculture.

10. Culinary Diversity: Plant-based cuisine encompasses a wide range of culinary traditions from around the world, offering endless possibilities for exploration and creativity in the kitchen.

11. Adaptability: Plant-based main courses can be easily adapted to accommodate various dietary preferences and restrictions, including vegan, vegetarian, gluten-free, and soy-free diets.

12. Budget-Friendly: Plant-based ingredients such as beans, grains, and seasonal vegetables are often more affordable than animal products, making plant-based meals accessible to individuals on a tight budget

Lean Proteins and Fish Recipes

Let's delve into the realm of lean proteins and fish, highlighting their significance in a cancer-fighting diet. Lean proteins provide essential amino acids for cellular repair and muscle maintenance, while fish offer a rich source of omega-3 fatty acids, known for their anti-inflammatory properties. From succulent grilled salmon to savoury lentil burgers, these recipes strike a balance between flavour and nutrition, making them ideal choices for individuals seeking to optimise their health and well-being.

1. High-Quality Protein: Lean proteins, such as chicken breast, turkey, tofu, and legumes, are rich in high-quality protein, essential for supporting muscle growth, repair, and overall body function.

2. Amino Acid Profile: Lean proteins provide a complete amino acid profile, ensuring that your body has all the building blocks necessary for synthesising proteins and supporting various physiological processes.

3. Satiety: Protein-rich meals promote feelings of fullness and satiety, helping to control appetite and prevent overeating, which can aid in weight management and reduce the risk of obesity-related cancers.

4. Low in Saturated Fat: Lean proteins are low in saturated fat and cholesterol, making them heart-healthy choices that support cardiovascular health and reduce the risk of heart disease, a common comorbidity of cancer.

5. Omega-3 Fatty Acids: Fish, such as salmon, mackerel, and sardines, are rich sources of omega-3 fatty acids, which have anti-inflammatory properties and may help reduce the risk of cancer progression and recurrence.

6. Brain Health: Omega-3 fatty acids are crucial for brain health and cognitive function, supporting memory, concentration, and mood stability.

7. Heart Health: Consuming fish regularly is associated with a lower risk of heart disease and stroke, attributed to the cardioprotective effects of omega-3 fatty acids, which help lower blood pressure, reduce triglyceride levels, and prevent plaque buildup in the arteries.

8. Versatility: Lean proteins and fish can be prepared in a variety of ways, including grilling, baking, sautéing, and steaming, allowing for endless culinary creativity and versatility in the kitchen.

9. Sustainable Seafood: Choosing sustainably sourced fish helps protect marine ecosystems and fish populations, ensuring that future generations can continue to enjoy the benefits of seafood consumption.

10. Vitamin D: Fatty fish like salmon and tuna are excellent sources of vitamin D, which plays a role in immune function, bone health, and cancer prevention.

11. Iron and Zinc: Lean proteins such as poultry and legumes provide essential minerals like iron and zinc, which are important for immune function, wound healing, and overall health.

12. Plant-Based Options: For those following a vegetarian or vegan diet, plant-based sources of protein like tofu, tempeh, lentils, and chickpeas offer nutritious alternatives to animal products.

Cancer-Fighting Side Dishes

Let's delve into the realm of side dishes designed to complement your main meals while offering a powerhouse of nutrients and cancer-fighting potential. These side dishes are not only flavorful and satisfying but also packed with a diverse array of vitamins, minerals, antioxidants, and phytochemicals known for their protective effects against cancer. From vibrant roasted vegetables to hearty whole grain salads, each recipe is crafted to elevate your dining experience while nourishing your body from within. By incorporating these cancer-fighting side dishes into your meals, you'll not only tantalise your taste buds but also take proactive steps towards supporting your overall health and well-being.

1. Abundance of Vegetables: Cancer-fighting side dishes are often centred around an abundance of colourful vegetables, providing a spectrum of vitamins, minerals, and phytonutrients essential for optimal health and cancer prevention.

2. Fibre-Rich Ingredients: Whole grains, legumes, and vegetables found in these side dishes are rich in dietary fibre, which promotes digestive health, regulates blood sugar levels, and may lower the risk of colorectal cancer.

3. Antioxidant Power: Many ingredients used in cancer-fighting side dishes are rich in antioxidants, which help neutralise harmful free radicals, reduce oxidative stress, and protect cells from damage that can lead to cancer development.

4. Anti-Inflammatory Properties: Certain foods featured in these side dishes, such as leafy greens, berries, nuts, and seeds, are known for their anti-inflammatory properties, which can help reduce chronic inflammation linked to cancer and other diseases.

5. Low in Added Sugars and Processed Ingredients: Cancer-fighting side dishes prioritise whole, minimally processed ingredients while minimising added sugars, refined grains, and unhealthy fats commonly found in processed foods, promoting overall health and well-being.

6. Balanced Macronutrients: These side dishes are often well-balanced in macronutrients, providing a combination of carbohydrates, protein, and healthy fats to support energy levels, satiety, and overall nutrition.

7. Variety of Cooking Methods: Cancer-fighting side dishes can be prepared using a variety of cooking methods, including roasting, steaming, sautéing, and grilling, allowing for versatility in flavour and texture.

8. Seasonal Ingredients: Many recipes in this category utilise seasonal ingredients, ensuring freshness, flavour, and nutritional quality while also supporting local agriculture and sustainability efforts.

9. **Meal Enhancement:** These side dishes serve as the perfect complement to main courses, adding depth of flavour, texture, and nutritional value to your meals while enhancing the overall dining experience.

10. **Family-Friendly Options:** Whether you're cooking for yourself, your family, or guests, cancer-fighting side dishes offer family-friendly options that appeal to a wide range of tastes and preferences, making them suitable for any occasion.

11. **Meal Prep Friendly:** Many of these side dishes can be prepared in advance and stored for later use, making meal planning and preparation more convenient and efficient.

12. **Creative Culinary Expression:** Cancer-fighting side dishes inspire creativity in the kitchen, encouraging you to experiment with new ingredients, flavours, and culinary techniques to create delicious and nutritious meals.

Balanced Dinner Plates

Creating a balanced dinner plate is essential for ensuring your body receives the nutrients it needs for optimal health and cancer prevention. Here are some guidelines for crafting a nutritious dinner plate.

1. Vegetables: Aim to cover at least half of your plate with a variety of colourful vegetables, such as leafy greens, cruciferous vegetables (broccoli, cauliflower, Brussels sprouts), bell peppers, carrots, or squash. Vegetables provide essential vitamins, minerals, and antioxidants that support overall health and reduce inflammation.

2. Whole Grains: Include a quarter of your plate with whole grains like quinoa, brown rice, whole-grain pasta, or whole-grain bread. Whole grains offer fibre, B vitamins, and other nutrients that support digestion and heart health.

3. Protein: Dedicate the remaining quarter of your plate to a healthy protein source like legumes, tofu, tempeh, fish, or lean poultry. Protein is essential for muscle repair, immune function, and maintaining a balanced diet.

4. Healthy Fats: Incorporate healthy fats like olive oil, avocado, nuts, or seeds into your meal for added flavour and nutrition. Healthy fats support brain function and help your body absorb fat-soluble vitamins.

5. Herbs and Spices: Season your meal with a variety of herbs and spices, like turmeric, garlic, ginger, basil, or rosemary, to add flavour and potential health benefits without the need for excessive amounts of salt, sugar, or unhealthy fats.

6. Colourful Fruits: While fruits may not always be a main feature on your dinner plate, consider adding a side of fresh berries, sliced melon, or a citrus salad for a boost of antioxidants and fibre.

7. Mindful Portioning: Pay attention to portion sizes and avoid overeating. Listen to your body's hunger and fullness cues to ensure you're consuming an appropriate amount of food for your individual needs.

8. Mediterranean-style dinner: featuring grilled eggplant, zucchini, and bell peppers, served with whole-grain pita and a Greek salad.
9. Stuffed bell peppers: filled with a mixture of quinoa, black beans, corn, and spices, served with a side of salsa and a green salad.

10. Vegetable stir-fry: with edamame, bell peppers, broccoli, and carrots, served over soba noodles with a light soy-based sauce. These balanced dinner plate ideas incorporate a variety of cancer-fighting ingredients while offering delicious and satisfying meals for you to enjoy.

Some balanced dinner plate examples include
1 Grilled salmon, roasted vegetables (broccoli, bell peppers, and carrots), and quinoa.
2 Tofu stir-fry with brown rice, mixed vegetables, and a light soy-ginger sauce.
3 Lentil and sweet potato curry with a side of whole-grain pita and a mixed green salad.

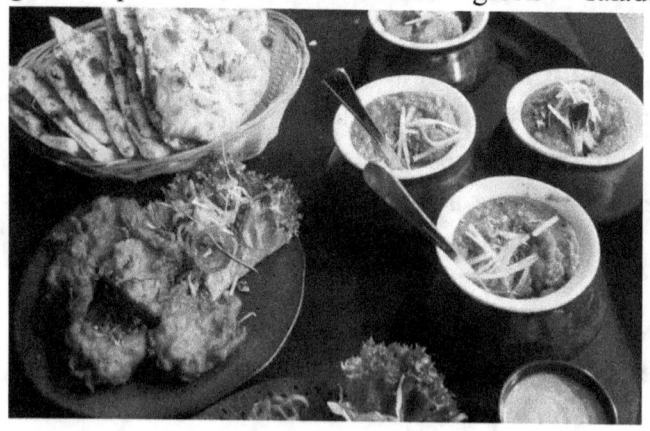

Chapter 7: Snacks and Small Bites

Quick and Healthy Snacks

Let's dive into the world of quick and healthy snacks, offering a plethora of options to satisfy your cravings while nourishing your body. These snacks are designed to provide a burst of energy and satiety between meals, without compromising on taste or nutrition. From crunchy vegetable sticks with hummus to homemade trail mix and Greek yoghourt parfaits, each snack is carefully crafted to deliver a combination of protein, fibre, healthy fats, and essential nutrients. Whether you're looking for a mid-morning pick-me-up or a post-workout refuel, these snacks are convenient, delicious, and sure to keep you fueled and satisfied throughout the day.

1. Nutrient Density: Quick and healthy snacks are packed with nutrients, including vitamins, minerals, antioxidants, and phytonutrients, providing a nutrient-dense option to support overall health and well-being.

2. Portion Control: These snacks are portion-controlled to help prevent overeating and promote mindful eating habits, making them an ideal choice for those looking to manage their weight or maintain portion control.

3. Satiety: Incorporating protein, fibre, and healthy fats into snacks helps promote feelings of fullness and satiety, keeping hunger at bay and preventing excessive snacking throughout the day.

4. Energy Boost: Quick and healthy snacks provide a quick energy boost to help combat fatigue and keep you alert and focused throughout the day, making them perfect for busy schedules and hectic lifestyles.

5. Blood Sugar Management: Snacks with a balanced combination of carbohydrates, protein, and fats can help stabilise blood sugar levels, preventing energy crashes and reducing the risk of cravings and overeating.

6. Convenience: These snacks are convenient and portable, making them easy to grab on the go or pack for work, school, or travel, ensuring that healthy choices are always within reach.

7. Versatility: Quick and healthy snacks come in a variety of flavours and textures, from sweet to savoury, crunchy to creamy, allowing for endless variety and customization to suit individual tastes and preferences.

8. Homemade Options: Many snacks can be prepared ahead of time or made from scratch using simple, wholesome ingredients, giving you control over the quality and nutritional content of your snacks.

9. Budget-Friendly: Making snacks at home can be more cost-effective than purchasing pre-packaged options, helping you save money while also reducing waste and environmental impact.

10. Gut Health: Some snacks, such as yoghurt with probiotics or fibre-rich fruits and vegetables, support gut health and digestion, promoting a healthy microbiome and overall digestive function.

11. Hydration: Snacks like fresh fruits and vegetables contribute to hydration, providing additional fluids and electrolytes to support hydration levels and overall hydration status.

12. Stress Relief: Enjoying a satisfying snack can help alleviate stress and anxiety, providing a moment of relaxation and enjoyment amidst a busy day.

Anti-Cancer Dips and Spreads

Dips and spreads can be a great addition to an anti-cancer diet when they're made with nutritious ingredients. Here are some delicious and healthy dip and spread ideas to incorporate into your meal plan.

1. Hummus: A Middle Eastern dip made from mashed chickpeas, tahini (sesame seed paste), lemon juice, garlic, and olive oil. It's high in protein and fibre, and provides essential vitamins and minerals. Chickpeas are a good source of plant-based protein, which contributes to satiety and muscle health, while tahini adds heart-healthy monounsaturated fats.

2. Guacamole: A creamy, avocado-based dip that's rich in heart-healthy monounsaturated fats, fiber, potassium, and various vitamins. Avocados contain antioxidants like oleuropein and hydroxytyrosol, which have anti-inflammatory properties and may help reduce the risk of some types of cancer.

3. Tzatziki: A Greek yoghurt-based dip with cucumber, garlic, and herbs. It's a good source of protein, calcium, and probiotics, which support gut health and digestion. Greek yoghurt also provides vitamin D, which has been linked to a reduced risk of cancer.

4. Black Bean Dip: A fibre-rich dip made from black beans, lime juice, cumin, and cilantro. Black beans are packed with fibre, protein, and antioxidants, which help maintain stable blood sugar levels and promote heart health. This dip is a great alternative to traditional hummus and pairs well with wholegrain pita or fresh vegetables.

5. Roasted Eggplant and Garlic Spread: Roasted eggplant and garlic are blended with olive oil, lemon juice, and tahini to create a flavorful and nutrient-dense spread. Eggplant contains anthocyanins, which have anti-inflammatory and anti-cancer properties, while garlic has been shown to have immune-boosting and antimicrobial effects.

6. Edamame Dip: A protein-packed dip made from edamame, lemon juice, garlic, and olive oil. Edamame is a good source of plant-based protein, fibre, and antioxidants, which support overall health and contribute to satiety.

7. Spinach and Artichoke Dip: A creamy and flavorful dip made with spinach, artichoke hearts, Greek yoghurt, and a touch of Parmesan cheese. Spinach is rich in iron, vitamins A and C, and antioxidants, while artichokes provide fibre and may help lower cholesterol levels.

8. Pesto: A vibrant green spread made from fresh basil, pine nuts, Parmesan cheese, garlic, and olive oil. Pesto is a good source of healthy fats, vitamins, and minerals, and it pairs well with pasta dishes, sandwiches, or as a vegetable dip.

9. Tapenade: A savoury spread made from olives, capers, anchovies, garlic, and olive oil. Olives are rich in monounsaturated fats, vitamin E, and polyphenols, which possess antioxidant properties that may help protect against cellular damage.

10. Roasted Red Pepper and Walnut Dip: A flavorful spread made from roasted red peppers, walnuts, garlic, and olive oil. Red peppers are high in vitamins A and C, as well as antioxidants like lycopene and beta-carotene, while walnuts provide omega-3 fatty acids that promote heart health and support cognitive function.

11. White Bean and Rosemary Dip: A smooth and creamy dip made from cannellini beans, fresh rosemary, lemon juice, and olive oil. White beans provide fibre and plant-based protein, which support digestive health and satiety.

12. Pumpkin and Sage Spread: A festive dip made from roasted pumpkin, fresh sage, garlic, and Greek yoghurt. Pumpkin is rich in beta-carotene, fibre, and potassium, while sage contains compounds that may improve brain function and have anti-inflammatory properties.

Nutritious Bars and Bites

Let's delve into the realm of nutritious bars and bites, offering a variety of options to satisfy your cravings while providing a boost of energy and nutrition. These bars and bites are designed to be convenient, portable, and packed with wholesome ingredients to fuel your body on the go. From homemade granola bars and energy balls to nut butter spreads and fruit-based bites, each snack is crafted to deliver a balance of carbohydrates, protein, healthy fats, fibre, and essential nutrients. Whether you need a quick pick-me-up between meals, a pre- or post-workout snack, or a healthy treat to satisfy your sweet tooth, these nutritious options are sure to keep you energised and satisfied throughout the day.

1. Balanced Nutrition: Nutritious bars and bites are formulated to provide a balanced combination of macronutrients, including carbohydrates, protein, and healthy fats, to support sustained energy levels and satiety.

2. Convenience: These snacks are convenient and portable, making them ideal for on-the-go lifestyles, busy schedules, and travel, ensuring that you always have a nutritious option within reach.

3. Quick Energy: With their blend of carbohydrates and natural sugars from ingredients like fruits, nuts, and seeds, these snacks provide a quick energy boost to fuel your body and brain, making them perfect for busy days or when you need a pick-me-up.

4. Satiety: Incorporating protein, fibre, and healthy fats into bars and bites helps promote feelings of fullness and satiety, preventing excessive snacking and reducing the risk of overeating.

5. Controlled Portions: Pre-portioned bars and bites help prevent overeating and promote mindful eating habits, making them an ideal choice for those looking to manage their weight or practice portion control.

6. Homemade Option: Many bars and bites can be made at home using simple, wholesome ingredients, giving you control over the quality and nutritional content of your snacks while allowing for customization to suit your taste preferences.

7. Variety: From chewy granola bars to crunchy energy bites, there's a wide variety of textures and flavours to choose from, ensuring that there's something for everyone's palate and preferences.

8. Customization: Homemade bars and bites can be customised with a variety of add-ins, such as nuts, seeds, dried fruits, and spices, allowing you to tailor them to your nutritional needs and flavour preferences.

9. Allergen-Friendly Options: Many recipes can be adapted to accommodate common dietary restrictions and allergies, such as gluten-free, dairy-free, nut-free, and vegan diets, ensuring inclusivity and accessibility for all.

10. Cost-Effective: Making bars and bites at home can be more cost-effective than purchasing pre-packaged options, helping you save money while also reducing waste and environmental impact.

11. Hydration: Some recipes incorporate hydrating ingredients like dried fruits and coconut, contributing to overall hydration levels and supporting optimal hydration status throughout the day.

12. Gut Health: Snacks made with ingredients like nuts, seeds, and whole grains provide fibre and prebiotics that support gut health and digestion, promoting a healthy microbiome and regular bowel movements.

Portable Snacks for On-the-Go

Let's delve into the world of portable snacks, offering a wide array of options that are perfect for busy lifestyles, travel, work, school, or any time you're on the move. These snacks are designed to be convenient, packable, and easy to enjoy wherever life takes you. From single-serve packs of nuts and seeds to fruit bars, jerky, veggie sticks, and more, each snack is carefully chosen to provide a balance of nutrients, flavours, and textures to keep you fueled and satisfied throughout your day. Whether you need a quick energy boost between meetings, a healthy snack for a road trip, or a satisfying treat for a hike or outdoor adventure, these portable options are sure to keep you nourished and energised no matter where your day takes you.

1. Convenience: Portable snacks are designed to be convenient and easy to grab on the go, making them perfect for busy schedules, travel, or anytime you need a quick bite.

2. Packability: These snacks come in individual or resealable packaging, making them easy to pack in a purse, backpack, or lunchbox without worrying about spills or messes.

3. Long Shelf Life: Many portable snacks have a long shelf life, making them ideal for stocking up and keeping on hand for whenever hunger strikes.

4. Variety: There's a wide variety of portable snacks to choose from, including sweet and savoury options, crunchy and chewy textures, and flavours to suit every palate.

5. Nutrient Dense: Despite their small size, portable snacks are often packed with nutrients, including protein, fibre, vitamins, and minerals, to keep you fueled and satisfied between meals.

6. Satiety: Snacks with a balance of protein, fibre, and healthy fats help keep you feeling full and satisfied, preventing overeating and reducing the risk of unhealthy food choices later on.

7. Energy Boost: Portable snacks provide a quick energy boost to help combat fatigue and keep you focused and alert throughout the day.

8. Portion Control: Snack packs and single-serve options help prevent overeating and promote portion control, making them an excellent choice for those watching their calorie intake or managing their weight.

9. Hydration: Many portable snacks, such as fruit bars or freeze-dried fruits, contribute to hydration levels, providing additional fluids and electrolytes to support overall hydration status.

10. Allergen-Friendly Options: There are plenty of allergen-friendly options available, including nut-free, gluten-free, dairy-free, and vegan snacks, ensuring that everyone can find something suitable for their dietary needs.

11. Kid-Friendly: Portable snacks are perfect for kids' lunchboxes, after-school snacks, or on-the-go adventures, providing a convenient and nutritious option for busy families.

12. Cost-Effective: Buying snacks in bulk or in multipacks can be more cost-effective than purchasing single-serving options, saving you money in the long run.

Chapter 8: Desserts with Benefits

Guilt-Free Sweet Treats

In this chapter, we delve into the world of guilt-free sweet treats, offering delicious and satisfying options that satisfy your sweet tooth without compromising your health goals. These treats are carefully crafted to provide indulgence without the guilt, using wholesome ingredients and smart substitutions to reduce added sugars, unhealthy fats, and empty calories. From decadent desserts made with nutrient-rich ingredients to creative twists on classic favourites, each recipe is designed to prove that you can enjoy sweets while still prioritising your health. Whether you're craving chocolate, cookies, cakes, or other sweet delights, these guilt-free treats offer a satisfying solution that nourishes your body and satisfies your cravings.

1. Nutrient-Rich Ingredients: Guilt-free sweet treats are made with nutrient-rich ingredients such as whole grains, nuts, seeds, fruits, and natural sweeteners, providing essential vitamins, minerals, and antioxidants to support overall health.

2. Reduced Added Sugars: These treats are sweetened with natural alternatives like honey, maple syrup, or dates, reducing the amount of refined sugars and preventing blood sugar spikes.

3. Healthy Fats: Many guilt-free sweet treats incorporate healthy fats from sources like nuts, seeds, and avocado, providing satiety and promoting heart health.

4. High in Fiber: With ingredients like whole grains, fruits, and nuts, these treats are high in fiber, supporting digestive health and helping you feel full and satisfied.

5. Lower in Calories: Compared to traditional sweets, guilt-free treats often contain fewer calories per serving, making them a lighter option for those watching their calorie intake.

6. Balanced Macronutrients: These treats are carefully balanced with carbohydrates, protein, and fat, providing sustained energy and preventing sugar crashes.

7. Gluten-Free Options: Many guilt-free sweet treats offer gluten-free variations for those with sensitivities or dietary preferences.

8. Vegan-Friendly: With plant-based ingredients, these treats are suitable for vegans and vegetarians, offering inclusive options for all dietary lifestyles.

9. Allergen-Free Alternatives: Recipes often include allergen-free alternatives for common allergens like dairy, eggs, nuts, and soy, ensuring that everyone can enjoy these treats safely.

10. Simple and Easy to Make: Despite their health-conscious ingredients, these treats are simple and easy to make, requiring minimal time and effort in the kitchen.

11. Kid-Friendly Options: Guilt-free sweet treats are perfect for kids' snacks or lunchbox treats, providing a healthier alternative to store-bought sweets.

12. Customizable Recipes: Many recipes are customizable, allowing you to adjust ingredients to suit your taste preferences or dietary needs.

Anti-Cancer Baking

Let's venture into the realm of anti-cancer baking, where the act of baking meets the science of cancer prevention. Here, we reimagine traditional baking recipes by incorporating ingredients rich in cancer-fighting properties, ensuring that every bite contributes to your overall health and well-being. From antioxidant-packed desserts to fiber-rich bread alternatives, each recipe is thoughtfully designed to harness the healing power of food and promote a lifestyle that supports cancer prevention and recovery. By embracing anti-cancer baking, you not only nourish your body but also cultivate a deeper understanding of how simple culinary choices can play a significant role in your journey towards optimal health.

1. Incorporating Anti-Inflammatory Ingredients: Anti-cancer baking recipes often feature ingredients known for their anti-inflammatory properties, such as turmeric, ginger, and cinnamon, which can help combat chronic inflammation linked to cancer development.

2. Rich in Antioxidants: These recipes prioritise ingredients rich in antioxidants, such as berries, dark chocolate, and nuts, which help neutralise free radicals and protect cells from damage that may lead to cancer.

3. Whole Grain Alternatives: Instead of refined flours, anti-cancer baking utilises whole grain flours like whole wheat, spelt, or oat flour, providing fibre and essential nutrients that support digestive health and reduce cancer risk.

4. Natural Sweeteners: Recipes often rely on natural sweeteners like honey, maple syrup, or dates instead of refined sugars, offering sweetness without the negative health effects associated with excessive sugar consumption.

5. Healthy Fats: Incorporating sources of healthy fats such as avocado, olive oil, and nuts adds richness and texture to baked goods while providing essential fatty acids that support heart health and reduce inflammation.

6. Nutrient-Dense Additions: Ingredients like flaxseeds, chia seeds, and hemp seeds are commonly included in anti-cancer baking recipes for their high nutrient content, including omega-3 fatty acids, fiber, and protein.

7. Low Glycemic Index Options: Using ingredients with a low glycemic index helps regulate blood sugar levels and insulin response, reducing the risk of insulin resistance and related cancers.

8. Inclusion of Herbs and Spices: Herbs and spices like rosemary, thyme, and oregano are often incorporated into anti-cancer baking for their potent antioxidant and anti-inflammatory properties.

9. Dairy-Free and Plant-Based Variations: Many recipes offer dairy-free and plant-based alternatives to traditional dairy products, accommodating individuals with lactose intolerance or following a vegan diet.

10. Gluten-Free Options: For those with gluten sensitivities or celiac disease, anti-cancer baking recipes often include gluten-free flour alternatives like almond flour, coconut flour, or gluten-free oats.

11. Focus on Digestive Health: Ingredients like psyllium husk, flaxseed meal, and fermented foods promote gut health and may reduce the risk of certain cancers by supporting a healthy microbiome.

12. Balanced Nutrient Profile: Anti-cancer baking recipes aim for a balanced nutrient profile, ensuring that each treat provides a mix of carbohydrates, protein, and fat to support overall health and energy levels.

Fruit-Based Desserts

Let's delve into the world of fruit-based desserts, where nature's bounty takes centre stage in creating delicious and health-conscious sweet treats. From vibrant fruit salads to decadent fruit tarts, each recipe celebrates the natural sweetness and nutritional richness of fruits while offering a guilt-free indulgence. By embracing fruit-based desserts, you not only satisfy your sweet cravings but also nourish your body with an array of vitamins, minerals, and antioxidants essential for optimal health and cancer prevention.

1. Abundance of Vitamins and Minerals: Fruit-based desserts are packed with essential vitamins and minerals, including vitamin C, potassium, and folate, which support immune function, heart health, and overall well-being.

2. Antioxidant Powerhouse: Fruits are rich in antioxidants such as flavonoids, polyphenols, and vitamin E, which help combat oxidative stress and reduce the risk of cancer and other chronic diseases.

3. Fibre-Rich Delights: With their high fiber content, fruit-based desserts promote digestive health, regulate blood sugar levels, and contribute to satiety, making them a nutritious choice for satisfying cravings.

4. Low-Calorie Options: Many fruit-based desserts are naturally low in calories and fat, making them suitable for those watching their weight or managing conditions like diabetes.

5. Versatility of Flavors and Textures: From juicy berries to creamy avocado, fruit-based desserts offer a diverse range of flavours and textures, allowing for endless creativity in recipe development.

6. Natural Sweetness: Fruits provide natural sweetness without the need for added sugars, offering a healthier alternative to traditional desserts while satisfying the palate.

7. Hydration Benefits: Fruits with high water content, such as watermelon and cucumbers, help keep the body hydrated and support optimal functioning of bodily systems.

8. Seasonal Variety: Fruit-based desserts can be tailored to the seasons, showcasing the best of each season's harvest and ensuring freshness and flavour.

9. Immune-Boosting Properties: Certain fruits, such as citrus fruits and kiwi, are rich in vitamin C, known for its immune-boosting properties that help protect against infections and support wound healing.

10. Heart-Healthy Options: Fruits like berries, grapes, and apples contain compounds that support heart health by reducing inflammation, lowering cholesterol levels, and improving blood vessel function.

11. **Brain-Boosting Nutrients:** Blueberries, in particular, are renowned for their cognitive benefits, thanks to their high levels of antioxidants and flavonoids that support brain health and may reduce the risk of age-related cognitive decline.

12. **Digestive Support:** Fruits like papaya and pineapple contain enzymes such as papain and bromelain, which aid in digestion and may alleviate digestive discomfort.

Indulgent Yet Healthy Puddings

Let's dive into the world of indulgent yet healthy puddings, where velvety textures and rich flavours meet nutritious ingredients to create desserts that delight the senses while supporting your well-being. From creamy chia seed puddings to luscious avocado chocolate mousse, each recipe strikes the perfect balance between decadence and nutritional value. Indulge guilt-free as you discover how these wholesome puddings can satisfy your sweet cravings while fueling your body with essential nutrients for optimal health and vitality.

1. Creaminess without Compromise: Indulgent yet healthy puddings offer the luxurious texture and richness of traditional desserts without relying on heavy creams or excessive sugars, providing a guilt-free indulgence.

2. Nutrient-Dense Ingredients: These puddings are crafted with nutrient-dense ingredients such as avocados, chia seeds, coconut milk, and cacao, which are rich in vitamins, minerals, antioxidants, and healthy fats essential for overall health and disease prevention.

3. Omega-3 Boost: Puddings featuring chia seeds, flaxseeds, or hemp seeds are excellent sources of omega-3 fatty acids, known for their anti-inflammatory properties and benefits for heart and brain health.

4. Fibre-Rich Delicacies: Many pudding recipes incorporate high-fibre ingredients like fruits, nuts, seeds, and whole grains, promoting digestive health, regulating blood sugar levels, and supporting weight management.

5. Blood Sugar Balance: By using natural sweeteners like maple syrup, honey, or dates in moderation, these puddings offer a lower glycemic load compared to traditional desserts, helping to maintain stable blood sugar levels.

6. **Antioxidant Power:** Puddings featuring ingredients like dark chocolate, berries, and matcha provide a potent dose of antioxidants that help neutralise free radicals, protect cells from damage, and reduce the risk of chronic diseases.

7. **Dairy-Free Options:** Many recipes are dairy-free, making them suitable for individuals with lactose intolerance or dairy sensitivities while still offering a creamy and satisfying texture.

8. **Allergy-Friendly Varieties:** Indulgent yet healthy puddings can easily accommodate various dietary restrictions and preferences, including gluten-free, vegan, and paleo diets, ensuring inclusivity and accessibility for all.

9. **Mood-Boosting Ingredients:** Cacao-based puddings contain compounds like theobromine and phenylethylamine, which may enhance mood, increase serotonin levels, and promote feelings of happiness and well-being.

10. **Hydration Support:** Puddings made with coconut milk or fruit purees contribute to hydration

and electrolyte balance, providing a refreshing and nourishing option, especially in warmer climates.

11. Post-Workout Recovery: Puddings containing ingredients like bananas, nuts, and seeds offer a convenient post-workout snack, providing essential nutrients for muscle repair, replenishing glycogen stores, and promoting recovery.

12. Brain-Boosting Benefits: Ingredients like avocados and walnuts are rich in monounsaturated fats and antioxidants that support brain health, cognitive function, and may reduce the risk of neurodegenerative diseases.

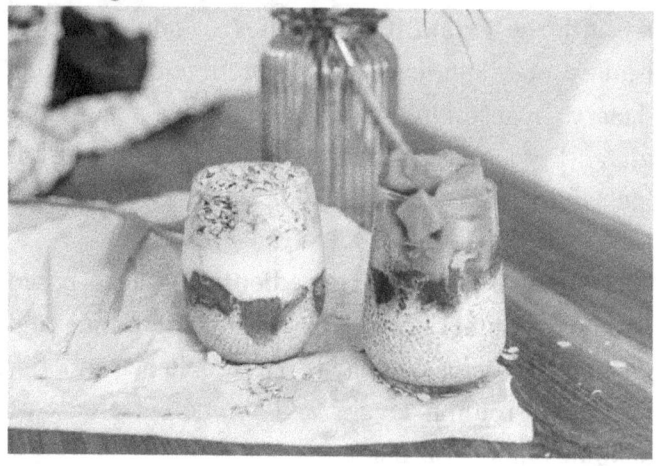

Chapter 9: Beverages That Heal

Anti-Inflammatory Teas

In the realm of holistic health, few beverages rival the comforting embrace and healing potential of anti-inflammatory teas. This chapter delves into the world of these aromatic concoctions, where ancient wisdom meets modern science to deliver a symphony of flavours and therapeutic benefits. From the gentle warmth of turmeric-infused blends to the invigorating zest of ginger-laced brews, each cup offers a journey of rejuvenation and renewal for both body and soul.

1. Nature's Pharmacy in a Cup: Anti-inflammatory teas harness the healing power of herbs, spices, and botanicals revered for their anti-inflammatory properties, providing a natural and holistic approach to wellness.

2. Turmeric's Golden Touch: Turmeric, with its active compound curcumin, takes centre stage in many anti-inflammatory teas, renowned for its potent anti-inflammatory and antioxidant effects, which may help alleviate pain, reduce inflammation, and support overall health.

3. Ginger's Warming Embrace: Ginger, prized for its spicy kick and therapeutic benefits, adds depth and warmth to teas, offering anti-inflammatory, digestive, and immune-boosting properties that promote vitality and well-being.

4. Soothing Chamomile: Chamomile tea, with its delicate floral aroma and gentle flavour, boasts anti-inflammatory and calming effects, making it a soothing remedy for stress, anxiety, and digestive discomfort.

5. Peppermint's Cooling Relief: Peppermint tea refreshes the senses with its cooling menthol flavour while providing anti-inflammatory and digestive support, soothing upset stomachs, and promoting relaxation.

6. Green Tea's Antioxidant Armour: Green tea, revered for its high concentration of antioxidants called catechins, offers potent anti-inflammatory properties that may help protect cells from damage, reduce inflammation, and support cardiovascular health.

7. Holy Basil's Sacred Nectar: Holy basil, or Tulsi tea, holds a revered place in Ayurvedic medicine for its adaptogenic and anti-inflammatory properties,

offering stress relief, immune support, and balance to mind, body, and spirit.

8. Cinnamon's Spicy Sweetness: Cinnamon tea delights the palate with its warm, spicy-sweet flavour while providing anti-inflammatory and antioxidant benefits, supporting blood sugar control, and enhancing heart health.

9. Rosehip's Floral Elegance: Rosehip tea, derived from the fruit of the rose plant, delivers a delicate floral flavour and a bounty of anti-inflammatory compounds like polyphenols and vitamin C, promoting immune health and skin rejuvenation.

10. Nettle's Nutrient-Rich Brew: Nettle tea, made from the leaves of the stinging nettle plant, offers a mineral-rich infusion with anti-inflammatory properties that may alleviate allergy symptoms, support joint health, and nourish the body.

11. Licorice's Sweet Soothing Symphony: Licorice tea, with its naturally sweet taste and medicinal properties, provides anti-inflammatory, digestive, and respiratory support, offering relief from sore throats, coughs, and gastrointestinal discomfort.

12. Hibiscus's Vibrant Vitality: Hibiscus tea delights with its bold crimson hue and tangy flavor,

delivering a burst of antioxidants and anti-inflammatory compounds that may help lower blood pressure, support heart health, and boost immune function.

Detoxifying Juices

Embark on a journey of rejuvenation and vitality with the vibrant world of detoxifying juices. This chapter delves into the refreshing realm of nutrient-packed elixirs, where fruits, vegetables, and herbs unite to cleanse the body, boost energy, and restore balance. From zesty citrus blends to verdant green concoctions, each glass brims with antioxidants, vitamins, and minerals, offering a delicious path to detoxification and renewal.

1. Nature's Cleansing Bount: Detoxifying juices harness the natural detoxifying properties of fruits, vegetables, and herbs, delivering a potent infusion of vitamins, minerals, and antioxidants that support the body's natural detoxification processes.

2. Citrus Sunshine: Citrus fruits like lemons, limes, and oranges take centre stage in many detoxifying juices, boasting high levels of vitamin C and antioxidants that promote immune health, aid digestion, and flush toxins from the body.

3. Green Goddess: Green juices, packed with nutrient-rich leafy greens like kale, spinach, and parsley, offer a verdant burst of chlorophyll, vitamins, and minerals that alkalize the body, support detoxification, and boost energy levels.

4. Roots of Renewal: Root vegetables such as carrots, beets, and ginger lend their earthy sweetness and detoxifying properties to juices, promoting liver health, improving digestion, and enhancing circulation.

5. Cleansing Herbs: Detoxifying juices often feature cleansing herbs like cilantro, parsley, and mint, prized for their ability to support liver function, eliminate heavy metals, and reduce inflammation throughout the body.

6. Hydrating Cucumber: Cucumber juice, with its high water content and refreshing flavour, hydrates the body, flushes out toxins, and supports skin health, making it an essential ingredient in detoxifying blends.

7. Tropical Paradise: Tropical fruits like pineapple, mango, and papaya infuse juices with exotic flavours and enzymatic activity that aids digestion, reduces inflammation, and promotes cellular detoxification.

8. Glowing Skin Elixirs: Juices rich in beta-carotene from carrots, sweet potatoes, and bell peppers nourish the skin from within, promoting a radiant complexion and protecting against oxidative stress and UV damage.

9. Green Tea Infusions: Green tea-based juices provide a double dose of detoxification with the antioxidant power of tea polyphenols and the cleansing properties of fresh fruits and vegetables, supporting overall health and vitality.

10. Alkalizing Lemongrass: Lemongrass, prized for its citrusy aroma and alkalizing effect, adds a refreshing twist to juices while supporting digestion, reducing inflammation, and promoting detoxification.

11. Ginger's Zesty Zing: Ginger juice, with its spicy kick and potent medicinal properties, invigorates the senses and aids digestion, making it a valuable addition to detoxifying blends for its anti-inflammatory and immune-boosting effects.

12. Beet's Blood-Purifying Power: Beet juice, with its deep red hue and earthy flavour, cleanses the blood, supports liver function, and boosts stamina and endurance, making it a staple ingredient in detoxifying juices for enhanced vitality.

Smoothies for Health

Indulge in a symphony of flavours and nutrients with the vibrant world of smoothies for health. This chapter is a celebration of wellness in a glass, where fruits, vegetables, superfoods, and supplements unite to create delicious and nutrient-rich concoctions. From revitalising breakfast blends to energising post-workout refuels, each smoothie offers a delectable way to fuel your body, support your immune system, and enhance your overall well-being.

1. Wholesome Nutrition on the Go: Smoothies provide a convenient and portable way to pack a myriad of nutrients into a single glass, making them ideal for busy lifestyles and on-the-go nourishment.

2. Fruitful Bounty: Fruits form the foundation of many smoothie recipes, offering a natural source of vitamins, minerals, fibre, and antioxidants that promote immune health, digestion, and overall vitality.

3. Green Elixirs: Green smoothies, enriched with leafy greens like spinach, kale, and Swiss chard, provide a powerful dose of chlorophyll, vitamins, and minerals that alkalize the body, support detoxification, and boost energy levels.

4. **Protein Powerhouses:** Protein-rich ingredients such as Greek yoghourt, nut butters, and protein powders add satiety and muscle-building benefits to smoothies, making them an excellent choice for post-workout recovery or meal replacement.

5. **Superfood Boosts:** Superfoods like chia seeds, flaxseeds, hemp hearts, and spirulina lend their nutritional prowess to smoothies, providing essential fatty acids, protein, antioxidants, and micronutrients that support overall health and well-being.

6. **Gut-Friendly Blends:** Probiotic-rich ingredients such as yoghourt, kefir, and fermented foods enhance gut health and digestion when incorporated into smoothies, promoting a balanced microbiome and immune function.

7. **Hydration Heroes:** Hydrating ingredients like coconut water, cucumber, and watermelon add refreshing hydration to smoothies, supporting optimal cellular function, electrolyte balance, and post-exercise recovery.

8. Energy-Boosting Blends: Smoothies infused with energizing ingredients like matcha green tea, maca powder, and bee pollen provide a natural source of sustained energy without the crash associated with caffeine or sugar-laden beverages.

9. Antioxidant-Rich Creations: Antioxidant-packed ingredients such as berries, cherries, and pomegranate seeds protect against oxidative stress, inflammation, and cellular damage, promoting overall health and longevity.

10. Immune-Enhancing Concoctions: Immune-boosting ingredients like citrus fruits, ginger, turmeric, and echinacea fortify the body's defences, supporting immune function and resilience against illness and infection.

11. Skin-Supportive Smoothies: Smoothies enriched with collagen peptides, vitamin C-rich fruits, and omega-3 fatty acids from flaxseeds or walnuts promote radiant skin, strong hair, and healthy nails from the inside out.

12. Detoxifying Blends: Detox smoothies featuring ingredients like beets, cilantro, and dandelion greens support liver detoxification, aid in the elimination of toxins, and promote overall cleansing and rejuvenation.

Hydrating and Healing Drinks

Embark on a journey of rejuvenation with a selection of hydrating and healing drinks designed to refresh the body, soothe the soul, and promote overall well-being. From revitalising elixirs to comforting tonics, each beverage offers a nourishing blend of ingredients aimed at hydrating the body, supporting detoxification, and enhancing vitality.

1. **Hydration at its Finest:** Hydrating drinks serve as a cornerstone of wellness, helping to replenish fluids lost throughout the day and maintain optimal hydration levels for overall health and vitality.

2. **Nourishing Elixirs:** Crafted with a variety of fruits, vegetables, herbs, and spices, hydrating drinks offer a potent source of vitamins, minerals, antioxidants, and phytonutrients that support cellular function and promote vitality.

3. **Electrolyte Replenishment:** Beverages enhanced with electrolyte-rich ingredients like coconut water, citrus fruits, and sea salt help restore electrolyte balance, making them ideal for rehydration after exercise or during hot weather.

4. **Detoxifying Tonics:** Detox drinks featuring ingredients such as lemon, ginger, and apple cider

vinegar support liver function, aid digestion, and promote the elimination of toxins from the body, helping to restore balance and vitality.

5. **Alkalizing Blends:** Alkaline drinks made with ingredients like cucumber, celery, and leafy greens help neutralise acidity in the body, promoting pH balance, reducing inflammation, and supporting overall health.

6. **Anti-Inflammatory Elixirs:** Beverages infused with anti-inflammatory ingredients such as turmeric, ginger, and green tea help reduce inflammation, soothe digestive discomfort, and support immune function.

7. **Adaptogenic Brews:** Adaptogenic drinks featuring herbs like ashwagandha, holy basil, and rhodiola help the body adapt to stress, support adrenal function, and promote resilience in the face of physical and emotional challenges.

8. **Gut-Supportive Tonics:** Beverages enriched with probiotics, prebiotics, and digestive enzymes help promote a healthy gut microbiome, support digestion, and enhance nutrient absorption for overall wellness.

9. Stress-Relieving Infusions: Calming drinks featuring ingredients like chamomile, lavender, and lemon balm help promote relaxation, reduce stress levels, and support mental and emotional well-being.

10. Sleep-Inducing Blends: Sleep-enhancing drinks made with ingredients such as valerian root, passionflower, and magnesium promote restful sleep, improve sleep quality, and support overall sleep hygiene.

11. Skin-Soothing Elixirs: Beverages enriched with collagen peptides, vitamin E, and antioxidant-rich fruits help promote skin health, hydration, and elasticity for a radiant complexion from the inside out.

12. Mindful Sips for Well-Being: Mindful drinking practices, such as savouring each sip, focusing on the sensory experience, and expressing gratitude for nourishment, enhance the enjoyment and therapeutic benefits of hydrating beverages.

Chapter 10: Meal Planning and Preparation

Creating an Anti-Cancer Meal Plan

Embark on a transformative journey toward vibrant health with a meticulously crafted anticancer meal plan designed to nourish your body, bolster your immune system, and support your overall wellbeing. By strategically selecting nutrient-rich foods and incorporating cancer-fighting ingredients into each meal, you'll lay the foundation for optimal health and resilience in the face of adversity.

1. Personalised Nutrition: Tailored to your unique dietary preferences, health goals, and nutritional needs, an anti-cancer meal plan provides a roadmap for making informed food choices that support your journey to wellness.

2. Whole Foods Foundation: Centred around whole, minimally processed foods, the meal plan emphasises the importance of incorporating a variety of fruits, vegetables, whole grains, lean proteins, and healthy fats to provide essential nutrients and phytochemicals that promote health and vitality.

3. Plant-Powered Plate: Plant-based foods take centre stage in the meal plan, providing a rich source of antioxidants, vitamins, minerals, and fibre that help reduce inflammation, support immune function, and combat oxidative stress – key factors in cancer prevention and treatment.

4. Colourful Variet: A rainbow of colours on your plate signifies a diverse array of nutrients, so the meal plan encourages incorporating a variety of colourful fruits and vegetables into your meals to maximise nutritional benefits and flavour profiles.

5. Lean Protein Sources: High-quality, lean protein sources such as poultry, fish, legumes, and tofu feature prominently in the meal plan, providing essential amino acids for muscle repair, immune function, and overall health.

6. Healthy Fats: Heart-healthy fats from sources like avocados, nuts, seeds, and olive oil are incorporated into the meal plan to support brain health, hormone production, and nutrient absorption, while also providing satiety and flavour.

7. Mindful Portion Control: The meal plan emphasises mindful eating practices, including paying attention to hunger and fullness cues, practising portion control, and savouring each bite to promote optimal digestion and satisfaction.

8. Balanced Macronutrients: Each meal is thoughtfully balanced to include a combination of carbohydrates, protein, and fat, providing sustained energy, stable blood sugar levels, and a feeling of satisfaction throughout the day.

9. Strategic Meal Timing: The meal plan incorporates strategic meal timing to optimise energy levels, support digestion, and promote metabolic health, with an emphasis on regular meals and snacks spaced evenly throughout the day.

10. Hydration Support: Adequate hydration is essential for overall health and well-being, so the meal plan includes recommendations for hydrating beverages and encourages drinking water throughout the day to stay properly hydrated.

11. Cancer-Fighting Ingredients: Key anti-cancer ingredients such as cruciferous vegetables, berries, turmeric, garlic, green tea, and mushrooms are strategically incorporated into the meal plan to provide powerful antioxidants, phytochemicals, and other bioactive compounds that promote cellular health and resilience.

12. Seasonal and Local Produce: Whenever possible, the meal plan encourages the use of seasonal and locally sourced produce to maximise freshness, flavour, and nutrient content while supporting local farmers and sustainable agriculture practices.

Batch Cooking and Freezing Tips

Streamline your meal preparation process and ensure access to nourishing meals at any time with these batch cooking and freezing tips tailored to your anticancer meal plan. By dedicating a few hours to cooking in advance and utilising proper storage techniques, you'll save time, reduce food waste, and effortlessly maintain a healthy eating routine, even on your busiest days.

1. Strategic Meal Selection: Choose recipes that lend themselves well to batch cooking, such as soups, stews, casseroles, and grain-based dishes, which can be easily scaled up and portioned for later use.

2. Planning and Organization: Before you begin cooking, take inventory of your ingredients, plan your meals for the week, and create a shopping list to ensure you have everything you need on hand.

3. Efficient Cooking Process: Maximise efficiency by multitasking in the kitchen – for example, while a soup simmers on the stove, you can prep vegetables for roasting or chop ingredients for a salad.

4. **Large-Batch Preparation:** Prepare larger quantities of your favourite recipes to yield multiple servings, making it easy to portion out meals for the week ahead.

5. **Portion Control:** After cooking, portion out individual servings of your meals into freezer-safe containers or resealable bags to prevent overeating and make it convenient to grab a meal whenever hunger strikes.

6. **Labelling and Dating:** Clearly label each container with the name of the dish and the date it was prepared to keep track of freshness and ensure that you use up older meals first.

7. **Freezing Techniques:** For optimal freshness and flavour, allow cooked dishes to cool completely before transferring them to the freezer. Consider investing in high-quality freezer-safe containers or vacuum-sealed bags to minimise the risk of freezer burn and preserve food quality.

8. **Flat Freezing Method:** Lay flat freezer bags or containers on a baking sheet to freeze individual

portions in a uniform shape, making them easier to stack and store in the freezer.

9. Thawing Safely: When you're ready to enjoy a frozen meal, thaw it safely in the refrigerator overnight or use the defrost setting on your microwave to ensure even heating and prevent foodborne illness.

10. Reheating Tips: Reheat frozen meals in the microwave, on the stovetop, or in the oven until they reach a safe internal temperature, stirring occasionally or covering with a lid to prevent drying out.

11. Variety and Rotation: Maintain a diverse selection of frozen meals to prevent taste fatigue and ensure you always have options that appeal to your cravings and dietary preferences.

12. Emergency Meals: Keep a selection of pre-portioned frozen meals on hand for busy days, unexpected guests, or times when you're too tired to cook, providing a convenient and nutritious alternative to takeout or processed foods.

Balancing Nutrients Throughout the Day

Maintaining a well-balanced diet rich in essential nutrients is key to supporting your body's natural defences against cancer. Learn how to strategically incorporate a variety of nutrients into your daily meals to optimise your health and enhance your body's ability to fight off disease. By focusing on nutrient density, portion sizes, and meal timing, you can create a balanced eating pattern that nourishes your body from sunrise to sunset.

1. **Foundational Nutrients:** Start your day with a nutritious breakfast that includes a balance of macronutrients carbohydrates, proteins, and healthy fats to provide sustained energy and support overall well-being.

2. **Protein Power:** Incorporate lean proteins such as poultry, fish, tofu, or legumes into each meal to promote muscle repair, satiety, and immune function.

3. **Whole Grain Goodness:** Choose whole grains like quinoa, brown rice, or whole wheat bread to provide complex carbohydrates, fibre, and essential vitamins and minerals for lasting energy and digestive health.

4. Vibrant Veggies: Aim to fill half of your plate with colourful vegetables at each meal to boost your intake of antioxidants, vitamins, and minerals while adding flavour and texture to your dishes.

5. Leafy Greens: Include leafy greens such as spinach, kale, or Swiss chard in your meals to increase your consumption of cancer-fighting phytonutrients like chlorophyll and carotenoids.

6. Healthy Fats: Incorporate sources of healthy fats such as avocado, nuts, seeds, and olive oil into your meals to support brain health, hormone production, and inflammation control.

7. Balanced Snacking: Choose nutrient-dense snacks such as Greek yoghourt with fruit, whole grain crackers with hummus, or a handful of nuts to curb hunger between meals and prevent overeating later in the day.

8. Hydration Habits: Stay hydrated throughout the day by drinking water, herbal teas, and other hydrating beverages to support digestion, circulation, and detoxification.

9. Mindful Eating: Practise mindful eating by paying attention to hunger and fullness cues, savouring each bite, and avoiding distractions to prevent overeating and promote digestive wellness.

10. Meal Timing: Aim to eat regular meals and snacks spaced evenly throughout the day to maintain stable blood sugar levels, prevent energy crashes, and support optimal metabolism.

11. Nutrient Density: Choose foods that are nutrient-dense meaning they provide a high concentration of vitamins, minerals, and antioxidants relative to their calorie content to maximise the nutritional value of your meals.

12. Variety and Moderation: Embrace variety in your diet by incorporating a wide range of foods from all food groups while practising moderation and portion control to maintain a healthy balance of nutrients.

Sample Weekly Menus

Take the guesswork out of meal planning with these sample weekly menus designed to support your anti-cancer journey. Each day features a balanced selection of nutrient-rich meals and snacks, showcasing the delicious variety and flexibility of an anti-cancer diet. From hearty breakfasts to satisfying dinners, these menus provide a roadmap for nourishing your body and promoting optimal health.

Monday
Breakfast: Energising Smoothie with spinach, banana, berries, almond milk, and protein powder.
Lunch: Superfood Salad with mixed greens, grilled chicken breast, quinoa, avocado, cherry tomatoes, and balsamic vinaigrette.
Snack: Carrot sticks with hummus.
Dinner: Baked salmon with roasted Brussels sprouts and sweet potatoes.

Tuesday
Breakfast: Overnight oats with Greek yogurt, mixed berries, chia seeds, and honey.
Lunch: Curried lentil soup with whole grain bread and a mixed green side salad.
Snack: Apple slices with almond butter.
Dinner: Mediterranean-style quinoa bowls with lemon-garlic shrimp, roasted vegetables (bell peppers, zucchini, and eggplant), cherry tomatoes, feta cheese, and a drizzle of olive oil.

Wednesday:
Rise and Shine: Wake up to an Anti-Cancer Breakfast Bowl filled with Greek yogurt, fresh berries, and crunchy granola, a delightful combination of flavours and textures.

Lunchtime Bliss: Dive into a Hearty Lentil Soup brimming with nutrient-dense vegetables and hearty legumes, a comforting and satisfying meal for a busy day.
Midday Munch: Enjoy the satisfying crunch of whole grain crackers topped with creamy almond butter, a simple yet nourishing snack to keep you fueled.
Dinner Delight: Indulge in the warmth and flavour of Lean Turkey Chili served with a side of whole grain cornbread, a cosy and satisfying meal for a relaxing evening.

Thursday:
Breakfast: Healthy Morning Beverage, Green tea with lemon and honey.
Lunch: Anti-Cancer Sandwich, Whole grain bread with grilled chicken, lettuce, tomato, avocado, and mustard.
Snack: Sliced cucumbers with tzatziki sauce.
Dinner: Plant-Based Main Course, Lentil and vegetable curry served over brown rice.

Friday:
Breakfast: Greek yoghourt parfait with granola, sliced strawberries, and a drizzle of honey.
Lunch: Superfood Wrap with whole wheat tortilla, hummus, grilled vegetables, feta cheese, and spinach.

Snack: Mixed nuts and dried fruit.

Dinner: Balanced Dinner Plate, Grilled shrimp skewers with quinoa pilaf and steamed asparagus.

Saturday:
Breakfast: Anti-Cancer Breakfast Bowl, Acai bowl topped with granola, sliced banana, and shredded coconut.
Lunch: Superfood Salad, Quinoa salad with arugula, roasted beets, goat cheese, and walnuts.
Snack: Apple slices with almond butter.
Dinner: Lean Proteins and Fish Recipe, Baked cod with lemon herb sauce, served with roasted potatoes and green beans.

Sunday:
Breakfast: Nutrient-Packed Omelette, Spinach, tomato, and feta cheese omelette with whole grain toast.
Lunch: Hearty Vegetable Soup with barley, carrots, celery, and kale, served with whole grain crackers.
Snack: Cottage cheese with pineapple chunks.
Dinner: Plant-Based Main Course, Mushroom and lentil stuffed bell peppers with a side of quinoa.

Chapter 11: Dining Out and Social Events

Making Smart Choices at Restaurants

Eating out can be a challenge when you're trying to maintain an anti-cancer diet. However, with some strategic choices and a bit of planning, you can enjoy dining out while still adhering to your health goals. Eating out often means less control over ingredients and cooking methods, which can lead to higher intake of unhealthy fats, sugars, and processed foods. By making mindful choices, you can enjoy meals that support your health and wellness. Here's a comprehensive guide to help you make smart choices at restaurants.

1. Research the Menu Ahead of Time: Look up the restaurant's menu online before you go. Many restaurants offer nutritional information which can help you plan your meal in advance.

2. Choose Restaurants with Healthy Options: Opt for places known for their healthy menus, such as those offering farm-to-table, organic, or whole foods. Ethnic cuisines like Japanese, Mediterranean, and Indian often have plenty of healthy options.

3. Start with a Salad: Begin your meal with a salad loaded with colourful vegetables. Ask for the dressing on the side to control the amount you use. Avoid creamy dressings; opt for vinaigrettes instead.

4. Focus on Lean Proteins: Select dishes that feature lean proteins such as fish, chicken, or plant-based proteins like beans and lentils. Avoid fried or breaded proteins; go for grilled, baked, or steamed options.

5. Load Up on Vegetables: Ensure your plate is half-filled with vegetables. Steamed, roasted, or grilled veggies are excellent choices. Avoid vegetables cooked in heavy sauces or butter.

6. Choose Whole Grains: Opt for dishes that include whole grains like brown rice, quinoa, or whole-wheat pasta. These grains are high in fiber and essential nutrients.

7. Be Mindful of Portions: Restaurant portions can be large. Consider sharing a dish, ordering an appetiser as your main course, or immediately setting aside half of your meal to take home.

8. Stay Hydrated: Drink plenty of water before and during your meal. This can help you feel fuller and avoid overeating. Skip sugary drinks and opt for water, herbal teas, or sparkling water with lemon.

9. Skip Dessert or Choose Wisely: Restaurant desserts are often high in sugar and unhealthy fats. If you want something sweet, choose fruit or share a dessert with someone else.

10. Communicate with Your Server: Don't be afraid to ask your server about how dishes are prepared. Request modifications like grilling instead of frying or adding extra vegetables instead of bread.

11. Avoid All-You-Can-Eat Buffet: Buffets can encourage overeating and offer fewer healthy options. If you must eat at a buffet, start with a large salad and choose smaller portions of healthy foods.

12. Practise Mindful Eating: Eat slowly and savour each bite. Pay attention to your hunger and fullness cues, and stop eating when you're satisfied, not when you're stuffed.

Example Choices at Different Types of Restaurants

Italian: Choose grilled fish, minestrone soup, or a salad with a vinaigrette dressing. Skip the breadbasket and creamy pastas.

Mexican: Opt for grilled chicken or fish tacos on corn tortillas with plenty of vegetables. Avoid fried foods like chimichangas or nachos.

Chinese: Select steamed dumplings, vegetable stir-fries, or steamed fish. Limit dishes with heavy sauces or fried items like egg rolls.

American: Go for a grilled chicken salad, a veggie burger without the bun, or a lean steak with a side of vegetables. Skip the fries and sugary drinks.

Navigating Social Gatherings

Social gatherings, such as parties, family get-togethers, and celebrations, often revolve around food, which can make it challenging to maintain an anti-cancer diet. However, with a little planning and mindfulness, you can enjoy these events without compromising your health goals. Social events frequently feature foods that are high in unhealthy fats, sugars, and processed ingredients. By making thoughtful choices, you can enjoy the occasion while sticking to your anti-cancer dietary principles.

Tips for Navigating Social Gatherings

1. Eat Before You Go: Have a healthy meal or snack before attending a gathering. This can help you avoid arriving hungry and overindulging in less healthy options.

2. Bring a Healthy Dish: Offer to bring a dish to share. This ensures there will be at least one nutritious option available and can introduce others to delicious, healthy foods.

3. Survey the Options: Take a look at all the food choices before filling your plate. This allows you to make more informed decisions about what to eat.

4. Opt for Lean Proteins: Select lean protein options such as grilled chicken, fish, or plant-based proteins like beans and lentils. Avoid fried or breaded proteins.

5. Watch Your Portion: Use smaller plates if available and be mindful of portion sizes. It's okay to enjoy a variety of foods in moderation.

6. Limit Alcohol Consumption: Alcohol can be high in calories and can lower your inhibitions, leading to overeating. If you drink, choose red wine for its potential health benefits and limit yourself to one or two glasses.

7. Stay Hydrated: Drink plenty of water throughout the event. Staying hydrated can help control hunger and reduce the temptation to overeat.

8. Practise Mindful Eating: Eat slowly and savour your food. Pay attention to your hunger and fullness signals, and stop eating when you're satisfied.

9. Have a Plan for Desserts: If desserts are a part of the gathering, decide in advance how you will handle them. You can choose to have a small portion, share with someone, or opt for healthier dessert options like fruit.

10. Politely Decline Unhealthy Foods: It's okay to say no to foods that don't align with your dietary goals. Be polite but firm in your decisions, and don't feel pressured to eat something just to be polite.

Example Strategies for Different Types of Gatherings

Family Dinners: Offer to bring a healthy side dish or dessert. This ensures there's something you can eat and contributes to the meal.
Potlucks: Bring a dish that fits your dietary needs. Look for other healthy options that attendees have brought.
Work Events: Eat a healthy snack beforehand and stick to lighter options like salads and lean proteins. Avoid the dessert table if possible.

Festive Parties: Enjoy the festive foods in moderation. Choose smaller portions and fill up on healthier options first.

Bringing Your Own Anticancer Dishes

Bringing your own anticancer dishes to social gatherings is a proactive way to ensure you have healthy, nutritious options to enjoy. It also allows you to share the benefits of an anti-cancer diet with friends and family, potentially inspiring others to make healthier choices. Social gatherings often feature foods that may not align with an anti-cancer diet, such as those high in unhealthy fats, sugars, and processed ingredients. By bringing your own dishes, you can control what you eat and contribute to a more health-conscious atmosphere. Here are some advantages of embracing this practice.

1. Dietary Control: By bringing your own dishes, you have full control over the ingredients and preparation methods, ensuring that your food aligns with any dietary restrictions or preferences you may have.

2. Portion Control: Preparing your own meals allows you to manage portion sizes, supporting a healthier and more balanced diet.

3. Cost-effective: Bringing homemade dishes can save money compared to purchasing meals or takeout, as you can buy ingredients in bulk and cook larger quantities at once.

4. Environmental Impact: Using reusable containers and utensils reduces waste from disposable packaging and single-use items, contributing to a smaller ecological footprint.

5. Creative Outlet: Preparing your own dishes allows you to experiment with new recipes, ingredients, and cooking techniques, expanding your culinary horizons.

6. Share Cultural Dishes: By sharing homemade dishes at gatherings, you have the opportunity to introduce friends and colleagues to traditional or family recipes that they may not have experienced before.

7. Allergy Management: For those with food allergies or sensitivities, bringing your own dishes helps ensure that you have safe, allergen-free food options available.

8. Quality Ingredients: Preparing your own meals allows you to select high-quality, fresh ingredients that align with your nutrition goals and preferences. Bringing your own dishes is an excellent way to maintain a healthy, balanced diet while reducing environmental impact and promoting a sense of community through sharing delicious, homemade meals.

Tips for Bringing Anticancer Dishes

1. Plan Ahead: Consider the type of event and what dishes would be appropriate. Think about how the dish will be transported, served, and stored.

2. Choose Crowd-Pleasing Recipes: Opt for recipes that are universally appealing and familiar, but with a healthy twist. Think along the lines of salads, veggie platters, and whole grain dishes.

3. Focus on Fresh and Colourful Ingredients: Use a variety of colourful fruits and vegetables to make your dish visually appealing and packed with nutrients.

4. Balance Flavors and Textures: Create dishes that have a balance of flavours (sweet, savoury, tangy) and textures (crunchy, creamy) to make them more satisfying.

5. Prepare in Advance: Prepare as much as you can in advance to reduce stress on the day of the event. Some dishes, like salads or grain bowls, can be partially prepared and assembled just before serving.

6. Consider Dietary Needs of Others: Take into account any dietary restrictions of other guests, such as gluten-free or nut-free options, to ensure everyone can enjoy your dish.

7. Bring Enough for Sharing: Make enough so that others can taste and enjoy your healthy creation. This is an opportunity to showcase how delicious and satisfying healthy eating can be.

8. Label Your Dish: Include a small card with the name of the dish and key ingredients. This can help guests with allergies or dietary restrictions make informed choices.

9. Use Attractive Presentation: Presentation matters! Use attractive serving dishes and garnishes to make your dish look inviting and appetizing.

10. Share the Recipe: Be prepared to share the recipe with interested guests. Bringing a few printed copies or having a digital version ready to send can be a great way to spread healthy eating habits.

Example Anticancer Dishes to Bring

1. Quinoa Salad with Roasted Vegetable: A nutrient-dense salad featuring quinoa, a complete protein, and a mix of colourful roasted vegetables.

2. Kale and Berry Salad: A vibrant salad with antioxidant-rich kale and berries, topped with a light vinaigrette.

3. Lentil and Veggie Soup: A hearty, warming soup packed with fibre and plant-based protein.

4. Stuffed Bell Peppers: Bell peppers filled with a mixture of whole grains, beans, and spices, baked until tender.

5. Hummus and Veggie Platter: Homemade hummus served with an array of fresh vegetables for dipping.

6. Fruit Skewers: Skewers of fresh fruit for a refreshing and easy-to-eat dessert.

7. Chickpea Salad Wrap: Whole grain wraps filled with a chickpea salad, avocado, and greens.

8. Sweet Potato and Black Bean Salad: A filling salad with roasted sweet potatoes, black beans, and a lime-cilantro dressing. portance of maintaining an anti-cancer diet while travelling, offers practical tips for various travel scenarios, and encourages a balanced, mindful approach to eating on the go.

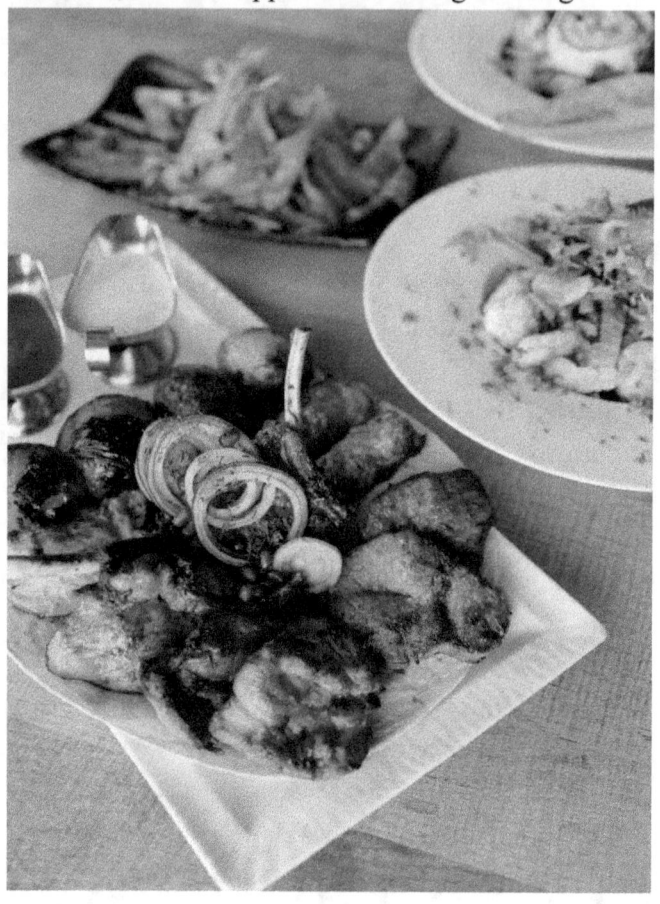

Chapter 12: The Mind-Body Connection

Stress Management and Cancer Prevention

Stress management plays a crucial role in cancer prevention and overall health. Chronic stress can weaken the immune system, increase inflammation, and lead to unhealthy behaviours, all of which can contribute to the development and progression of cancer. This section emphasises the importance of understanding and managing stress effectively.

1. Understanding Stress: Stress is the body's reaction to any change that requires an adjustment or response. It can be positive (eustress), like preparing for a wedding, or negative (distress), such as losing a job. Stress can be short-term (acute) or long-term (chronic).

2. Physiological Impact of Stress: Chronic stress leads to sustained high levels of stress hormones like cortisol and adrenaline. These hormones prepare the body for a "fight or flight" response but can be harmful if levels remain elevated over time, weakening the immune system and facilitating cancer cell growth.

3. Immune System Suppression: Chronic stress impairs the immune system, diminishing its ability to detect and destroy cancer cells. A weakened immune system leaves the body more susceptible to infections and diseases, including cancer.

4. Inflammation and Cancer: Stress triggers inflammation, a biological response to perceived threats. Chronic inflammation can promote the development and spread of cancer by creating an environment that supports tumour growth.

5. Behavioural Factors: Stress often leads to unhealthy behaviours like poor dietary choices, smoking, excessive alcohol consumption, and physical inactivity. These behaviours increase the risk of cancer and other chronic diseases.

6. Mindfulness and Meditation: Mindfulness and meditation practices help reduce stress by promoting relaxation and mental clarity. These techniques can lower cortisol levels, improve mood, and enhance overall well-being.

7. Physical Activities: Regular exercise is a potent stress reliever. Physical activity boosts the production of endorphins, which are natural mood elevators, and helps reduce levels of stress hormones.

Exercise also improves sleep quality and overall physical health.

8. Healthy Diet: A balanced diet supports overall health and helps stabilise mood and energy levels. Consuming anti-inflammatory foods, such as fruits, vegetables, whole grains, and omega-3 fatty acids, can mitigate the physical effects of stress.

9. Social Support: Building a strong support network of friends, family, and support groups provides emotional comfort and practical assistance. Social connections help reduce feelings of stress and isolation, offering a buffer against the negative effects of stress.

10. Professional Help: Professional help from therapists or counsellors can provide effective strategies for managing chronic stress and related mental health issues. Techniques such as cognitive-behavioural therapy (CBT) can help reframe negative thoughts and behaviours.

11. Incorporating Daily Practices: Incorporating stress management techniques into daily life can be simple yet effective. This includes setting aside time for relaxation, practising deep breathing exercises, engaging in hobbies, and ensuring regular physical activity.

12. Positive Mindset: Developing a positive outlook and practising gratitude can enhance resilience and reduce the perception of stress. Focusing on what you can control, celebrating small victories, and maintaining an optimistic attitude can significantly impact stress levels.

Incorporating Mindfulness into Meals

Understanding how diet influences cancer risk is essential for making informed choices about what we eat. Here's a detailed explanation of the link between diet and cancer .

1. Nutrient-Rich Foods: Foods rich in antioxidants, vitamins, minerals, and phytochemicals, such as fruits, vegetables, whole grains, and legumes, can help reduce the risk of cancer by protecting cells from damage and supporting a healthy immune system.

2. Processed and Red Meat: Consumption of processed and red meats has been linked to an increased risk of colorectal, pancreatic, and prostate cancers due to compounds that may damage cells and promote inflammation.

3. Sugary and Processed Foods: Diets high in sugary and processed foods, including snacks, desserts, and sugary beverages, are associated with a higher risk of breast, colorectal, and pancreatic cancers, contributing to weight gain, insulin resistance, and chronic inflammation.

4. Healthy Fats: Healthy fats found in olive oil, nuts, seeds, and fatty fish can lower the risk of certain cancers, including breast and prostate cancers, due to their anti-inflammatory properties and overall health benefits.

5. Alcohol Consumption: Excessive alcohol consumption is a known risk factor for various cancers, including those of the mouth, throat, oesophagus, liver, breast, and colon, as alcohol can damage cells and increase inflammation.

6. Fibre-Rich Foods: Diets high in fibre from fruits, vegetables, whole grains, and legumes can reduce the risk of colorectal cancer by promoting bowel regularity and reducing inflammation in the colon.

7. Calcium and Vitamin D: Adequate intake of calcium and vitamin D from foods or supplements may lower the risk of colorectal cancer by supporting cell growth regulation and immune function.

8. Mediterranean Diet: The Mediterranean diet, rich in fruits, vegetables, whole grains, fish, and olive oil, is associated with a reduced risk of cancer, including breast and colorectal cancers, due to its anti-inflammatory and antioxidant properties.

9. Plant-Based Diets: Vegetarian and vegan diets, emphasising plant foods while minimising or eliminating animal products, are linked to a lower risk of several cancers due to their high fiber, antioxidant, and phytochemical content.

10. Western Diet: The Western diet, high in red and processed meats, sugary and processed foods, and refined grains, is associated with an increased risk of cancer due to its promotion of inflammation, insulin resistance, and obesity.

11. Balance and Moderation: Overall dietary balance and moderation are essential for cancer prevention. No single food or nutrient can solely prevent or cause cancer, emphasising the importance of a diverse and balanced diet.

12. Informed Choices: Understanding the link between diet and cancer empowers individuals to make informed choices about their dietary habits, aiming to optimise health and reduce the risk of cancer and other chronic diseases.

Physical Activity and Nutrition

Understanding the interplay between physical activity and nutrition is crucial for maintaining overall health and preventing chronic diseases like cancer. Here's a comprehensive explanation.

1. Introduction to Physical Activity and Nutrition: Physical activity and nutrition are two pillars of a healthy lifestyle that work synergistically to promote overall well-being and reduce the risk of chronic diseases, including cancer.

2. Benefits of Physical Activity: Regular physical activity supports cardiovascular health, strengthens muscles and bones, enhances mood, and promotes better sleep quality.

Weight Management: Physical activity helps regulate body weight by burning calories and building lean muscle mass, which can reduce the risk of obesity-related cancers.

Reduced Cancer Risk: Engaging in regular physical activity has been linked to a lower risk of several types of cancer, including breast, colon, and prostate cancers, by improving immune function, reducing inflammation, and regulating hormone levels.

3. Types of Physical Activity

Aerobic Exercise: Activities such as walking, running, cycling, swimming, and dancing elevate heart rate and improve cardiovascular fitness.

Strength Training: Resistance exercises using weights or resistance bands help build muscle strength and endurance, improving overall physical function and metabolism.

Flexibility and Balance Exercises: Stretching and balance exercises improve flexibility, mobility, and coordination, reducing the risk of falls and injuries.

4. Role of Nutrition in Supporting Physical Activity: Proper nutrition provides the energy needed for physical activity while ensuring adequate nutrient intake for optimal health and performance.

Macronutrients: Carbohydrates, proteins, and fats are essential for fueling physical activity, repairing and building muscle tissue, and supporting overall metabolic function.

Micronutrients: Vitamins and minerals play crucial roles in energy metabolism, muscle function, and recovery after exercise. Adequate intake of vitamins and minerals from a balanced diet supports physical activity and exercise performance.

5. Pre-Exercise Nutrition: Consuming carbohydrates before exercise provides readily available energy for muscles and helps sustain performance during prolonged or intense workouts.

Proteins: Including protein before exercise supports muscle repair and growth, especially when combined with carbohydrates to enhance muscle glycogen replenishment.

Hydration: Adequate hydration before, during, and after exercise is essential for maintaining fluid balance, regulating body temperature, and supporting overall performance and recovery.

6. **Post-Exercise Nutrition:** Consuming a combination of protein and carbohydrates after exercise supports muscle recovery, replenishes glycogen stores, and enhances muscle protein synthesis.

Hydration: Replenishing fluids lost through sweat during exercise is crucial for preventing dehydration and supporting post-exercise recovery.

7. **Overall Dietary Guidelines for Physical Activity:** Emphasise a balanced diet rich in fruits, vegetables, whole grains, lean proteins, and healthy fats to provide essential nutrients for overall health and physical activity.

Portion Control: Practice portion control to ensure energy intake aligns with energy expenditure, maintaining a healthy weight and supporting physical activity goals.

Hydration: Drink plenty of water throughout the day and during exercise to stay hydrated and support optimal physical performance and recovery.

8. Lifestyle Integration: Find enjoyable and sustainable ways to incorporate physical activity into daily life, such as walking, cycling, gardening, or dancing.
Balancing Nutrition and Physical Activity: Strike a balance between nutrition and physical activity that aligns with individual preferences, goals, and lifestyle constraints.

9. Cancer Prevention Benefits of Physical Activity and Nutrition: Engaging in regular physical activity and maintaining a balanced diet can significantly reduce the risk of developing certain types of cancer, including breast, colon, and prostate cancers.
Mechanisms of Action: Physical activity and proper nutrition contribute to cancer prevention through various mechanisms, including reducing inflammation, supporting immune function, regulating hormone levels, and promoting healthy cell growth and repair.
Weight Management: Maintaining a healthy weight through physical activity and nutrition is crucial for cancer prevention, as obesity is a risk factor for several types of cancer.

Improved Overall Health: By supporting cardiovascular health, metabolic function, and mental well-being, physical activity and nutrition contribute to overall health and resilience against cancer and other chronic diseases.

10. **Challenges and Barriers:** Busy schedules and competing priorities can make it challenging to prioritise physical activity and healthy eating.

Access to Resources: Limited access to safe and affordable exercise facilities, fresh produce, and nutritious food options can hinder efforts to engage in physical activity and maintain a balanced diet.

Call Knowledge and Education: Lack of awareness or understanding of the importance of physical activity and nutrition for cancer prevention may prevent individuals from adopting healthy behaviours.

Cultural and Social Factors: Cultural norms, social influences, and community environments can impact dietary habits and physical activity levels, presenting both opportunities and barriers to healthy living.

11. **Strategies for Success:** Establish realistic and achievable goals for physical activity and nutrition, considering individual preferences, abilities, and lifestyle constraints.

Gradual Progression: Start with manageable changes and gradually increase physical activity levels and improve dietary habits over time to avoid burnout or injury.

Social Support: Seek support from friends, family members, or community groups to stay motivated and accountable for maintaining healthy behaviours.

Education and Resources: Access reliable information and resources on physical activity and nutrition, including reputable websites, books, and professional guidance from healthcare providers or registered dietitians.

Behavioural Strategies: Employ behavioural strategies such as self-monitoring, goal-setting, and positive reinforcement to sustain long-term adherence to healthy habits.

Adaptability: Be flexible and adaptable in finding ways to incorporate physical activity and nutritious eating into different environments, situations, and life stages.

12. Long-Term Sustainability: Lifestyle Approach: View physical activity and nutrition as integral components of a lifelong commitment to health and well-being, rather than short-term interventions.

Enjoyment and Variety: Choose activities and foods that are enjoyable, varied, and sustainable to maintain long-term adherence and prevent boredom or burnout.

Self-Care and Balance: Prioritise self-care, rest, and recovery alongside physical activity and nutrition to prevent burnout and promote overall well-being.

Consistency: Consistent adherence to healthy habits, even in the face of challenges or setbacks, is key to achieving long-term health benefits and cancer prevention.

Sleep and Recovery

Understanding the importance of sleep and recovery is important for maintaining overall health, well-being, and cancer prevention. Sleep and recovery are critical components of a healthy lifestyle that support physical, mental, and emotional well-being. Adequate sleep and effective recovery strategies are essential for optimizing performance, promoting recovery from physical activity, and reducing the risk of chronic diseases, including cancer. Here's a comprehensive explanation tailored for a wide audience.

1. **Physical Restoration:** During sleep, the body undergoes repair and restoration processes, including muscle growth, tissue repair, and immune system function.
Cognitive Function: Sleep plays a crucial role in cognitive processes such as memory consolidation, learning, and problem-solving, enhancing overall mental clarity and performance.

Emotional Regulation: Adequate sleep supports emotional regulation and resilience, reducing the risk of mood disorders such as depression and anxiety.

Hormonal Balance: Sleep influences hormone regulation, including those involved in appetite control, metabolism, and stress response, which are important for maintaining overall health.

2. **Recommended Sleep Duration:** The National Sleep Foundation recommends adults aim for 7-9 hours of sleep per night to support optimal health and well-being.

Sleep Quality : Quality of sleep is equally important as duration, with factors such as sleep depth, continuity, and efficiency impacting overall sleep quality.

3. **Physical Recovery:** Sleep is essential for physical recovery from exercise and daily activities, facilitating muscle repair, glycogen replenishment, and recovery of energy stores.

Mental and Emotional Recovery: Adequate sleep supports mental and emotional recovery by reducing stress, promoting emotional regulation, and enhancing mood and resilience.

4. **Impact of Poor Sleep on Healthy:** Increased Disease Risk, Chronic sleep deprivation and poor sleep quality are associated with an increased risk of

various chronic diseases, including obesity, diabetes, cardiovascular disease, and certain types of cancer.

Impaired Cognitive Function: Insufficient sleep can impair cognitive function, including memory, attention, and decision-making, negatively impacting overall performance and productivity.

Mood Disturbance: Sleep disturbances are linked to mood disorders such as depression and anxiety, affecting mental health and well-being.

5. MStrategies for Improving Sleep and Recovery: Maintain a consistent sleep schedule by going to bed and waking up at the same time each day, even on weekends.

Creating a Sleep-Friendly Environment: Create a comfortable sleep environment by minimising noise, light, and temperature disruptions and investing in a supportive mattress and pillows.

Limiting Stimulant: Reduce or eliminate stimulants such as caffeine and nicotine close to bedtime, as they can interfere with sleep quality.

Practising Relaxation Techniques: Engage in relaxation techniques such as deep breathing, meditation, or gentle stretching before bedtime to promote relaxation and prepare the body for sleep.

Managing Stress: Implement stress management strategies such as mindfulness, journaling, or engaging in hobbies to reduce stress levels and promote better sleep and recovery.

Prioritising Sleep Hygiene: Practise good sleep hygiene habits, such as avoiding screens before bedtime, limiting alcohol consumption, and creating a calming bedtime routine to signal to the body that it's time to wind down.

6. **Recovery Strategies Beyond Sleep:** Incorporate active recovery techniques such as light exercise, stretching, or foam rolling to promote circulation, reduce muscle soreness, and enhance recovery from physical activity.

Nutrition and Hydration: Support recovery with proper nutrition and hydration by consuming nutrient-rich foods and staying hydrated throughout the day.

Rest Days: Incorporate regular rest days into exercise routines to allow the body to recover and adapt to training stress, preventing overtraining and injury.

Stress Reduction: Minimise stressors in daily life through relaxation techniques, time management, and setting boundaries to support overall recovery and well-being.

7. **Individual Variability and Needs:** Recognize that individual sleep needs and recovery strategies may vary based on factors such as age, genetics, lifestyle, and overall health status.

Listening to Your Body: Pay attention to cues from your body regarding sleep needs and recovery status, adjusting behaviours and habits accordingly to support optimal health and performance. emotional recovery, allowing the brain to process emotions, memories, and experiences from the day.

8. **Sleep Hygiene:** Practising good sleep hygiene habits such as maintaining a consistent sleep schedule, creating a sleep-conducive environment, and avoiding stimulants before bedtime can help improve sleep quality.

Stress Management: Engaging in stress management techniques such as meditation, deep breathing, and yoga can improve sleep quality by promoting relaxation and reducing stress.

Exercise and Sleep: Regular physical activity can improve sleep quality, but it's important to avoid intense exercise too close to bedtime to prevent disruption to sleep.

Diet and Sleep: A balanced diet rich in whole, nutrient-dense foods can support sleep quality, while excessive caffeine, alcohol, or heavy meals close to bedtime can disrupt sleep patterns.

Sleep Disorders: Recognizing the signs of sleep disorders such as insomnia, sleep apnea, or restless leg syndrome is important, as these conditions can significantly impact sleep quality and overall health.

9. Napping: While short naps (20-30 minutes) can be beneficial for mood and alertness, excessive or irregular napping can disrupt nighttime sleep patterns.

10. Seeking Professional Help: If sleep problems persist despite implementing good sleep habits, seeking professional help from a healthcare provider or sleep specialist can be beneficial in identifying and treating any underlying issues.

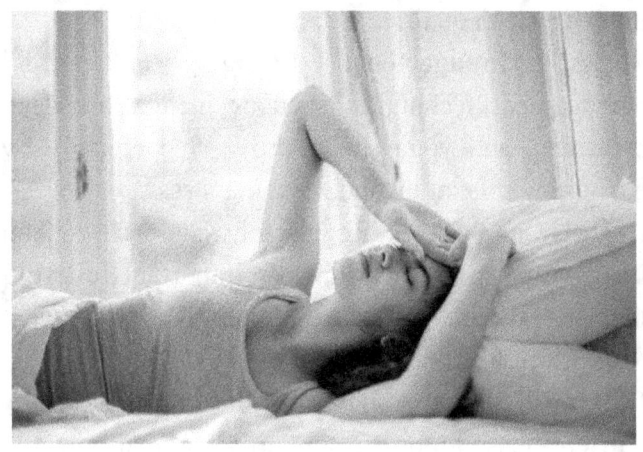

Chapter 13: Real-Life Success Stories

Inspiring Journeys of Cancer Survivors

"Inspiring Journeys of Cancer Survivors" captures the personal stories of individuals who have confronted cancer and emerged victorious. These narratives showcase the resilience, bravery, and perseverance of survivors, offering readers profound insight into the challenges and triumphs of the cancer journey. Through these real-life accounts, readers find hope, encouragement, and solidarity, recognizing the indomitable spirit that prevails in the face of adversity.

1. Real-life Stories, Jane's Triumph Over Breast Cancer: Jane was diagnosed with stage 2 breast cancer at the age of 42. Devastated but determined, she embraced a holistic approach to healing, focusing on nutrition, exercise, and stress management. Today, Jane is cancer-free and uses her experience to advocate for early detection and comprehensive cancer care.

2. Tom's Lifestyle Overhaul: Tom was diagnosed with prostate cancer at the age of 57. Motivated to make changes, he adopted a plant-based diet, began practising yoga, and prioritised sleep and self-care. Three years later, Tom is in remission and continues to inspire others with his passion for health and wellness.

3. Sarah's Journey with Ovarian Cancer: Sarah was diagnosed with ovarian cancer at just 28 years old. Combining traditional treatments with complementary therapies, such as acupuncture and mindfulness meditation, Sarah navigated her journey with grace and determination. Now cancer-free, she supports other young women facing cancer through mentorship and education.

4. Mike's Fight Against Colon Cancer: Mike was diagnosed with stage 3 colon cancer at age 37. Determined to beat the disease, he embraced a comprehensive approach that included targeted therapy, a health-promoting diet, and regular exercise. Today, Mike is in remission and shares his story to raise awareness about the importance of early detection and personalized cancer care.

2. Resilience and Courage: Survivors' stories vividly illustrate the incredible resilience and courage required to navigate the complexities of cancer diagnosis, treatment, and recovery, inspiring admiration and respect.

3. Triumph Over Adversity: Despite facing formidable challenges, survivors emerge victorious, celebrating triumphs both big and small along their journey, instilling hope and determination in others facing similar battles.

4. **Insight into the Cancer Journey:** Through survivors' narratives, readers gain a comprehensive understanding of the multifaceted nature of the cancer experience, including its physical, emotional, and psychological dimensions, fostering empathy and awareness.

5. **Unique Experiences:** Each survivor's story offers a unique perspective, reflecting the diversity of cancer experiences and emphasising the individuality of each journey, encouraging readers to appreciate the complexities and nuances of the cancer experience.

6. **Hope and Inspiration:** By sharing their stories of resilience and recovery, survivors offer a beacon of hope and inspiration to others facing cancer, demonstrating that healing and transformation are possible even in the face of adversity.

7. **Human Spirit:** Survivors' narratives illuminate the indomitable strength of the human spirit, highlighting the capacity for courage, perseverance, and resilience in overcoming life's greatest challenges, fostering admiration and awe.

8. Support and Positivity: The importance of support networks and maintaining a positive mindset is underscored in survivors' stories, emphasising the transformative power of love, encouragement, and optimism in the face of adversity.

9. Empathy and Solidarity: Readers are invited to empathise with survivors' struggles and triumphs, fostering a sense of solidarity and understanding within the cancer community, encouraging compassion and support for one another.

10. Coping Strategies: Survivors share practical coping strategies and insights they utilised to navigate the emotional and physical toll of cancer, offering valuable guidance and support to others on similar journeys, empowering readers with practical tools for resilience and adaptation.

How Diet Made a Difference

Diet plays a significant role in cancer prevention, treatment, and survivorship. This chapter highlights the transformative impact of dietary choices on individuals' cancer journeys, showcasing how nutrition can influence outcomes, enhance quality of life, and promote overall well-being.

1. Nutritional Influence: The chapter illuminates how dietary habits and choices can profoundly influence cancer risk, treatment response, and survivorship outcomes, emphasising the importance of nutrition in cancer care.

2. Prevention Strategies: Readers gain insights into dietary strategies for cancer prevention, including the consumption of antioxidant-rich foods, fibre, and phytochemicals, as well as the avoidance of processed foods, excess sugar, and unhealthy fats.

3. Supporting Treatment: Diet plays a crucial role in supporting individuals undergoing cancer treatment, providing essential nutrients to maintain strength, energy, and immune function while minimising side effects and enhancing treatment efficacy.

4. Managing Side Effects: Survivors share their experiences of using diet to manage treatment-related side effects such as nausea, fatigue, and appetite loss, offering practical tips and strategies for alleviating discomfort and improving quality of life.

5. Promoting Recovery: Post-treatment, survivors discuss how dietary modifications have supported their recovery journey, fostering healing, replenishing nutrient stores, and rebuilding strength and vitality.

6. **Optimising Long-term Health:** Diet plays a vital role in optimising long-term health and reducing the risk of cancer recurrence, with survivors adopting nutrient-rich, plant-based diets and embracing lifestyle changes to support ongoing wellness and vitality.

7. **Holistic Approach:** The chapter emphasises the importance of a holistic approach to nutrition, recognizing the interconnectedness of diet, physical activity, stress management, and overall lifestyle in promoting health and well-being.

8. **Personalised Nutrition:** Survivors highlight the value of personalised nutrition plans tailored to individual needs, preferences, and treatment histories, acknowledging the importance of working with healthcare professionals to optimise dietary choices.

9. **Educational Resources:** Readers are provided with access to educational resources, including cookbooks, meal plans, and online communities, to support them in making informed dietary decisions and navigating their cancer journey.

10. Mindful Eating: Survivors discuss the benefits of mindful eating practices, such as savouring each bite, listening to hunger and fullness cues, and cultivating a positive relationship with food, promoting a healthy and balanced approach to nutrition.

11. Culinary Creativity: The chapter celebrates culinary creativity and exploration, encouraging survivors to experiment with new recipes, flavours, and cooking techniques to make nutritious eating enjoyable and satisfying.

12. Family and Community Support: Survivors emphasise the importance of family and community support in adopting and maintaining healthy dietary habits, fostering a supportive environment conducive to wellness and recovery.

Practical Tips from Real People

In this chapter, real people who have navigated the challenges of cancer offer practical tips and insights garnered from their firsthand experiences. These tips cover a wide range of topics, from managing treatment side effects to maintaining emotional well-being and finding support. Let's delve deeper into each point.

1. **Managing Treatment Side Effects:** Survivors share strategies for coping with common treatment side effects like nausea, fatigue, and hair loss. Practical tips may include staying hydrated, eating small, frequent meals, and using cold caps during chemotherapy to minimise hair loss.

2. **Nutrition and Diet:** Real people offer advice on maintaining a balanced diet during treatment, emphasising the importance of nourishing foods to support the body's healing process. Tips may include incorporating nutrient-rich foods like fruits, vegetables, and lean proteins into meals and snacks.

3. **Exercise and Physical Activity:** Survivors highlight the benefits of staying active during treatment and beyond. Practical tips may include starting with gentle activities like walking or yoga, listening to your body's cues, and seeking guidance from a healthcare provider or physical therapist.

4. **Emotional Support:** Real people share strategies for managing the emotional toll of cancer, such as seeking support from loved ones, joining support groups, and practising self-care activities like meditation or journaling.

5. **Communication with Healthcare Providers:** Survivors stress the importance of open

communication with healthcare providers, including asking questions, expressing concerns, and advocating for personalised care.

6. Navigating the Healthcare System: Practical tips may include keeping organised records of appointments and treatments, understanding insurance coverage, and seeking assistance from patient navigators or social workers when needed.

7. Managing Finances: Real people offer advice on navigating the financial challenges of cancer, such as exploring resources for financial assistance, negotiating medical bills, and planning for unexpected expenses.

8. Maintaining Relationships: Survivors share strategies for maintaining relationships with family and friends during treatment, including setting boundaries, communicating openly, and seeking support from loved ones.

9. Self-Care Practices: Practical tips may include incorporating self-care practices into daily routines, such as mindfulness exercises, relaxation techniques, and hobbies that bring joy and fulfilment.

10. Setting Realistic Goals: Real people emphasise the importance of setting realistic goals and priorities during treatment, focusing on small accomplishments and milestones along the way.

11. Seeking Alternative Therapies: Survivors may share experiences with complementary and alternative therapies, such as acupuncture, massage therapy, or herbal supplements, and offer advice on integrating these approaches into overall care plans.

12. Spiritual and Religious Support: Practical tips may include seeking support from spiritual or religious communities, engaging in prayer or meditation, and finding solace in faith during difficult times.

Lessons Learned and Hope for the Future

In this chapter, individuals who have journeyed through cancer share the profound lessons they've gleaned from their experiences and offer hope for the future. Let's delve into these lessons and messages of hope.

1. Resilience in Adversity: Survivors reflect on their resilience in facing the challenges of cancer, emphasising the strength and courage they discovered within themselves during their journey.

2. Gratitude and Perspective: Individuals express gratitude for life's simple joys and newfound perspectives gained through their cancer experience, recognizing the importance of cherishing each moment and finding beauty in everyday life.

3. Acceptance and Surrender: Lessons learned include the power of acceptance and surrender in letting go of control and embracing uncertainty, allowing individuals to find peace and contentment amidst life's unpredictability.

4. Importance of Support: Survivors highlight the significance of support from family, friends, healthcare providers, and the broader cancer community, underscoring the healing power of connection and compassion in navigating the cancer journey.

5. Strength in Vulnerability: Lessons revolve around the strength found in vulnerability and the courage to share one's struggles and emotions openly, fostering deeper connections and understanding with others.

6. Mindfulness and Presence: Individuals discuss the practice of mindfulness and being present in the moment, cultivating awareness, gratitude, and inner peace amidst life's challenges and uncertainties.

7. Adaptability and Flexibility: Survivors share insights into the importance of adaptability and flexibility in adjusting to the ever-changing landscape of cancer treatment, recovery, and survivorship.

8. Finding Purpose and Meaning: Lessons learned include the journey of finding purpose and meaning in the face of adversity, discovering newfound passions, priorities, and opportunities for personal growth and fulfilment.

9. Resilience in Uncertainty: Individuals discuss resilience in navigating the uncertainty of life after cancer, embracing newfound perspectives, possibilities, and the resilience to face whatever the future may hold.

10. Hope and Optimism: Survivors offer messages of hope and optimism for the future, inspiring others to cultivate a positive outlook, resilience, and belief in the possibilities of healing, growth, and renewal.

Chapter 14: Special Considerations

Diet and Cancer Treatment Side Effects

Cancer treatments such as chemotherapy, radiation, and surgery can cause various side effects that impact a patient's appetite, digestion, and overall nutritional status. Proper dietary strategies are essential to help manage these side effects, improve quality of life, and support recovery. Cancer treatments can be physically and emotionally taxing, often leading to side effects that interfere with eating and nutrition. These side effects may include nausea, vomiting, diarrhoea, constipation, loss of appetite, taste changes, mouth sores, and fatigue. Proper nutrition can help mitigate these side effects, making it easier for patients to maintain their strength and health throughout treatment. Addressing each side effect with targeted dietary strategies can significantly improve a patient's quality of life and overall treatment outcomes. Detailed Points

1. Nausea and Vomiting: Frequent, Small Meal, Eating small, frequent meals throughout the day can help manage nausea. Large meals can be overwhelming and worsen symptoms.

Ginger: Incorporating ginger into your diet, such as ginger tea, ginger ale, or ginger candies, can help reduce nausea.

2. **Diarrhoea:** Staying hydrated is crucial. Drink clear fluids like water, broth, and electrolyte solutions to replace lost fluids.
Low-Fiber Foods: Opt for low-fibre foods like white rice, bananas, applesauce, and toast to help firm up stools and ease digestive distress.

3. **Constipation:** High-Fiber Foods, Incorporate high-fibre foods such as fruits, vegetables, whole grains, and legumes to promote regular bowel movements.
Hydration and Physical Activity: Drink plenty of water and engage in regular physical activity to support bowel function.

4. **Loss of Appetite:** Focus on nutrient-dense snacks like nuts, seeds, yoghourt, and cheese to ensure you're getting enough calories and nutrients even if your appetite is low.
Calorie-Rich Smoothies: Drink smoothies packed with fruits, vegetables, protein powder, and healthy fats to increase calorie intake without feeling overly full.

5. Taste Changes: Experiment with Flavors: Taste changes are common during treatment. Experiment with herbs, spices, marinades, and different cooking methods to find flavours that appeal to you.
Plastic Utensils: If you experience a metallic taste, try using plastic utensils instead of metal ones.

6. Mouth Sores: Eat soft, bland foods like mashed potatoes, smoothies, scrambled eggs, and yoghourt to avoid irritating mouth sores.
Avoid Irritants: Steer clear of spicy, acidic, or rough foods that can exacerbate mouth sores.

7. Fatigue: Balanced Meals: Consume balanced meals that include complex carbohydrates, lean proteins, and healthy fats to maintain energy levels.
Small, Frequent Meals: Eating smaller, more frequent meals can help sustain energy throughout the day.

8. Weight Loss: High-Calorie, High-Protein Foods, Include high-calorie, high-protein foods like avocados, nuts, seeds, cheese, and protein shakes to help maintain or gain weight.
Frequent Eating: Eat more frequently, focusing on nutrient-rich snacks and mini-meals.

9. Weight Gain: Whole, Unprocessed Foods, Focus on whole, unprocessed foods to manage weight gain.

Include plenty of fruits, vegetables, lean proteins, and whole grains.
Portion Control: Be mindful of portion sizes and avoid high-calorie, low-nutrient foods.

10. **Dry Mouth:** Sip water regularly and consider using saliva substitutes or sucking on ice chips.
Moist Foods: Choose moist foods like soups, stews, and casseroles to make swallowing easier.

11. **Difficulty Swallowing:** Puree foods or choose soft options like mashed potatoes, smoothies, and applesauce to ease swallowing difficulties.
Thickeners: Use commercial thickeners to adjust the consistency of liquids and prevent choking.

12. **Immune Support:** Eat a variety of nutrient-dense foods rich in vitamins, minerals, and antioxidants, such as berries, leafy greens, nuts, and seeds to support the immune system.
Probiotic: Include probiotic-rich foods like yoghurt, kefir, and fermented vegetables to support gut health and immunity.

Adjusting Your Diet Post-Diagnosis

Receiving a cancer diagnosis is life-altering, often necessitating significant changes in lifestyle, including diet. Post-diagnosis dietary adjustments are crucial in managing symptoms, enhancing treatment efficacy, and supporting overall well-being. After a cancer diagnosis, dietary adjustments become an integral part of the treatment and recovery process. Proper nutrition can help manage treatment side effects, boost the immune system, maintain strength and energy, and potentially improve treatment outcomes. Each person's nutritional needs may vary based on the type of cancer, stage, treatment plan, and individual health conditions. This section provides detailed guidance on tailoring your diet to meet these unique needs, ensuring that your body receives the nutrients it requires for optimal health during and after treatment.

1. Personalized Nutrition Plan: Work with a registered dietitian or nutritionist to develop a personalised nutrition plan tailored to your specific cancer type, treatment, and individual health needs.

Regular Monitoring: Adjust your diet based on regular health check-ups and nutritional assessments to address changing needs during treatment and recovery.

2. High Protein Intake: Include high-protein foods such as lean meats, fish, eggs, dairy products, legumes, nuts, and seeds to support muscle maintenance and repair.

Protein Supplements: Consider protein supplements if you struggle to meet your protein needs through food alone, especially during periods of low appetite.

3. Balanced Macronutrients: Opt for complex carbohydrates like whole grains, fruits, and vegetables for sustained energy and to support overall health.

Healthy Fats: Incorporate healthy fats from sources like avocados, nuts, seeds, and olive oil to provide essential fatty acids and support brain health.

4. Immune-Boosting Foods: Consume foods high in antioxidants, such as berries, leafy greens, and nuts, to help protect cells from damage and support immune function.

Probiotics: Include probiotic-rich foods like yogurt, kefir, and fermented vegetables to promote gut health and enhance the immune system.

5. Hydration: Ensure adequate hydration by drinking water, herbal teas, and clear broths. Proper hydration helps maintain bodily functions and manage treatment side effects like nausea and dry mouth.

Electrolyte Balance: Monitor and maintain electrolyte balance, especially if experiencing symptoms like vomiting or diarrhoea.

6. Small, Frequent Meals: Manage Appetite, Eat small, frequent meals throughout the day to manage appetite changes and maintain consistent nutrient intake.

Nutrient-Dense Snack: Choose nutrient-dense snacks, such as nuts, seeds, yogurt, and fruit, to ensure you're getting essential vitamins and minerals.

7. Managing Treatment Side Effects: Tailor your diet to manage specific treatment side effects like nausea, vomiting, diarrhoea, constipation, and taste changes, using strategies such as ginger for nausea or low-fibre foods for diarrhoea.

Soft and Bland Foods: Opt for soft and bland foods if experiencing mouth sores or difficulty swallowing to make eating more comfortable.

8. Anti-Inflammatory Foods: Include foods with anti-inflammatory properties, such as turmeric, ginger, fatty fish, and leafy greens, to help reduce inflammation and support recovery.

Avoid Pro-Inflammatory Food: Limit intake of processed foods, sugary drinks, and red meat, which can contribute to inflammation.

9. Supporting Digestive Healt: Maintain adequate fiber intake through fruits, vegetables, whole grains, and legumes to support digestive health and prevent constipation.

Probiotics and Prebiotics: Incorporate probiotics and prebiotics to promote a healthy gut microbiome, which is crucial for digestion and immune function.

10. **Energy Levels and Fatigue:** Consume balanced meals that include a mix of macronutrients to provide sustained energy and combat fatigue.

Iron-Rich Foods: Include iron-rich foods like lean meats, beans, and spinach to prevent anemia and support energy levels.

11. **Preventing Malnutrition:** Focus on nutrient-dense foods that provide essential vitamins and minerals, particularly if experiencing weight loss or reduced appetite.

Caloric Intake: Ensure adequate caloric intake to prevent malnutrition and maintain body weight, adjusting portions and food choices as needed.

12. **Stress and Emotional Eating:** Find healthy comfort foods that can help manage stress and emotional eating, such as dark chocolate, nuts, and whole grains.

Mindful Eating: Practise mindful eating techniques to stay aware of hunger and fullness cues, helping to manage emotional eating patterns.

Anti-Cancer Diets for Different Age Groups

A cancer diagnosis impacts individuals of all ages, and dietary needs can vary significantly based on age. From children to seniors, each age group has unique nutritional requirements that can support cancer treatment and overall health. The dietary needs of individuals can vary greatly across different stages of life. Children, adults, and seniors all require specific nutrients to support their growth, maintenance, and health, especially when dealing with cancer. This section aims to provide a detailed guide on how to adapt an anti-cancer diet for different age groups, ensuring that each individual receives the appropriate nutrients to support their immune system, manage treatment side effects, and promote overall well-being.

1. Infants and Toddlers: Breastfeeding Benefits, Emphasise the benefits of breastfeeding for infants, as it provides essential nutrients and antibodies that can strengthen the immune system.

Nutritious Weaning Foods: Introduce nutrient-dense foods like pureed vegetables, fruits, and grains when weaning, ensuring they receive vitamins and minerals crucial for growth and development.

2. Children (Ages 4-12): Balanced Diet, Ensure a balanced diet rich in fruits, vegetables, whole grains, lean proteins, and dairy to support growth and development.
Encouraging Healthy Eating Habits: Teach children about healthy eating habits, involving them in meal planning and preparation to foster a positive relationship with food.

3. Adolescents (Ages 13-18): High Nutrient Needs, Address the high nutrient needs of adolescents due to rapid growth and hormonal changes, focusing on calcium, iron, and protein intake.
Healthy Snacking: Encourage healthy snacking with options like fruits, nuts, and yoghourt to meet increased energy requirements and support overall health.

4. Young Adults (Ages 19-40): Maintaining Energy Levels, Focus on maintaining energy levels with a diet rich in complex carbohydrates, lean proteins, and healthy fats.
Lifestyle Integration: Integrate healthy eating into a busy lifestyle with easy-to-prepare, nutritious meals and snacks.

5. Middle-Aged Adults (Ages 41-60): Metabolism and Weight Management, Adjust caloric intake to match a potentially slowing metabolism, emphasising portion control and regular physical activity.

Chronic Disease Prevention: Include foods rich in antioxidants and anti-inflammatory properties to reduce the risk of chronic diseases.

6. Seniors (Ages 60+): Nutrient-Dense Foods, Prioritise nutrient-dense foods to ensure adequate intake of essential vitamins and minerals, as seniors may have decreased appetite.

Digestive Health: Focus on foods that are easy to digest and rich in fibre to support digestive health.

7. Cancer-Fighting Nutrients Across All Ages: Vitamins and Minerals, Ensure all age groups receive adequate vitamins (A, C, D, E) and minerals (calcium, magnesium, zinc) to support immune function and overall health.

Antioxidant-Rich Foods: Include a variety of antioxidant-rich foods like berries, leafy greens, and nuts to protect cells from damage.

8. Hydration: Adequate Fluid Intake: Emphasise the importance of staying hydrated across all age groups, as dehydration can exacerbate treatment side effects and hinder recovery.

9. Immune System Support: Immune-Boosting Foods, Incorporate immune-boosting foods like garlic, ginger, turmeric, and citrus fruits to enhance the body's ability to fight infections.

10. Managing Side Effects: Tailored Diets for Side Effects, Customise diets to manage common treatment side effects (nausea, vomiting, diarrhea) with appropriate food choices for each age group.

11. Maintaining Muscle Mass: Protein Intake: Ensure adequate protein intake to maintain muscle mass, especially in older adults, through sources like lean meats, legumes, and dairy.

12. Bone Health: Calcium and Vitamin D, Highlight the importance of calcium and vitamin D for bone health in children, adolescents, and seniors, using dairy products, leafy greens, and fortified foods.

Addressing Common Nutritional Deficiencies

Proper nutrition is crucial for overall health and well-being, especially during cancer treatment and recovery. Nutritional deficiencies can significantly impact a person's ability to withstand and recover from cancer therapy. Cancer patients are particularly vulnerable to nutritional deficiencies due to factors such as treatment side effects (nausea, vomiting, loss of appetite), the cancer itself interfering with nutrient absorption, and increased metabolic demands. This section aims to educate readers on identifying and addressing common nutritional deficiencies to ensure optimal health during and after cancer treatment. It covers essential nutrients, their roles in the body, signs of deficiency, and dietary sources to help mitigate these deficiencies.

1. Role of Vitamin D, Vitamin D: is vital for bone health and immune function. It helps the body absorb calcium, maintaining strong bones and teeth.

Signs of Deficiency: Symptoms include bone pain, muscle weakness, and an increased risk of fractures.

Sources of Vitamin D: Obtain vitamin D from sunlight exposure, fatty fish (salmon, mackerel), fortified dairy products, and supplements if necessary.

2. Role of Calcium: Calcium is critical for bone health, nerve function, and muscle contraction.

Signs of Deficiency: Symptoms include muscle cramps, weak or brittle nails, and an increased risk of osteoporosis.

Sources of Calcium: Include dairy products (milk, cheese, yoghourt), leafy green vegetables (kale, broccoli), fortified plant-based milks, and almonds.

3. **Role of Vitamin B12:** Vitamin B12 is important for nerve function, red blood cell production, and DNA synthesis.

Signs of Deficiency: Symptoms include fatigue, weakness, constipation, loss of appetite, and neurological issues like numbness or tingling.

Sources of Vitamin B12: Obtain from animal products (meat, fish, dairy), fortified cereals, and B12 supplements, especially for vegetarians and vegans.

4. **Folate (Vitamin B9):** Role of Folate, Folate is crucial for DNA synthesis and repair, and for producing healthy red blood cells.

Signs of Deficiency: Symptoms include fatigue, mouth sores, poor growth, and changes in skin, hair, or fingernail colour.

Sources of Folate: Include dark green leafy vegetables, legumes, nuts, seeds, and fortified grains.

5. **Role of Protein:** Protein is essential for tissue repair, muscle maintenance, and immune function.

Signs of Deficiency: Symptoms include muscle wasting, fatigue, and weakened immune response.

Sources of Protein: Incorporate lean meats, poultry, fish, eggs, dairy products, legumes, nuts, and seeds.

6. **Role of Magnesium:** Magnesium is involved in over 300 biochemical reactions in the body,

including muscle and nerve function, blood glucose control, and bone health.
Signs of Deficiency: Symptoms include muscle cramps, mental disorders, osteoporosis, fatigue, and high blood pressure.
Sources of Magnesium: Include nuts, seeds, whole grains, leafy green vegetables, and fortified foods.

7. **Role of Zinc:** Zinc is important for immune function, wound healing, DNA synthesis, and cell division.
Signs of Deficiency: Symptoms include weakened immune response, hair loss, diarrhea, and delayed wound healing.
Sources of Zinc: Include meat, shellfish, legumes, seeds, nuts, and dairy products.

8. **Role of Omega-3s:** Omega-3 fatty acids are important for brain function, reducing inflammation, and heart health.
Signs of Deficiency: Symptoms include dry skin, depression, poor concentration, and joint pain.
Sources of Omega-3s: Include fatty fish (salmon, mackerel, sardines), flaxseeds, chia seeds, walnuts, and fish oil supplements.

9. **Role of Fibre:** Fibre is important for digestive health, blood sugar control, and reducing cholesterol levels.

Signs of Deficiency: Symptoms include constipation, blood sugar fluctuations, and increased cholesterol levels.

Sources of Fibre: Include fruits, vegetables, whole grains, legumes, nuts, and seeds.

10. **Role of Vitamin A:** Vitamin A is crucial for vision, immune function, and skin health.

Signs of Deficiency: Symptoms include night blindness, dry skin, and increased susceptibility to infections.

Sources of Vitamin A: Include liver, fish oils, milk, eggs, and orange or yellow vegetables like carrots and sweet potatoes.

11. **Role of Vitamin C:** Vitamin C is important for the growth and repair of tissues, immune function, and antioxidant protection.

Signs of Deficiency: Symptoms include scurvy, characterised by fatigue, gum inflammation, and skin issues.

Sources of Vitamin C: Include citrus fruits, strawberries, bell peppers, broccoli, and Brussels sprouts.

12. **Role of Potassium:** Potassium is essential for muscle function, nerve signalling, and maintaining fluid balance.

Signs of Deficiency: Symptoms include muscle weakness, cramping, fatigue, and heart palpitations.

Sources of Potassium: Include bananas, oranges, potatoes, spinach, and legumes.

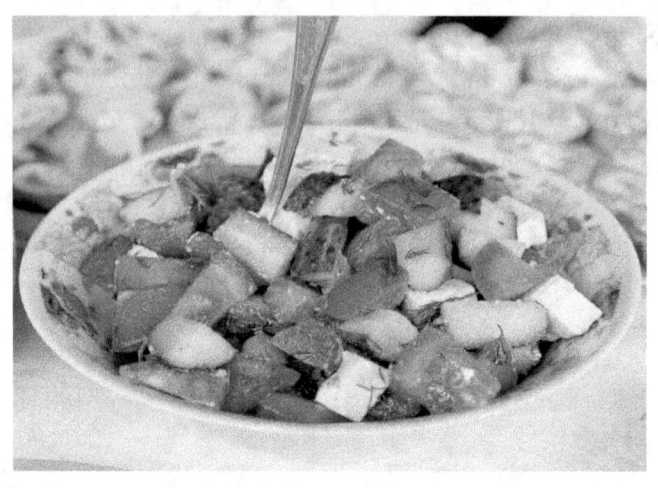

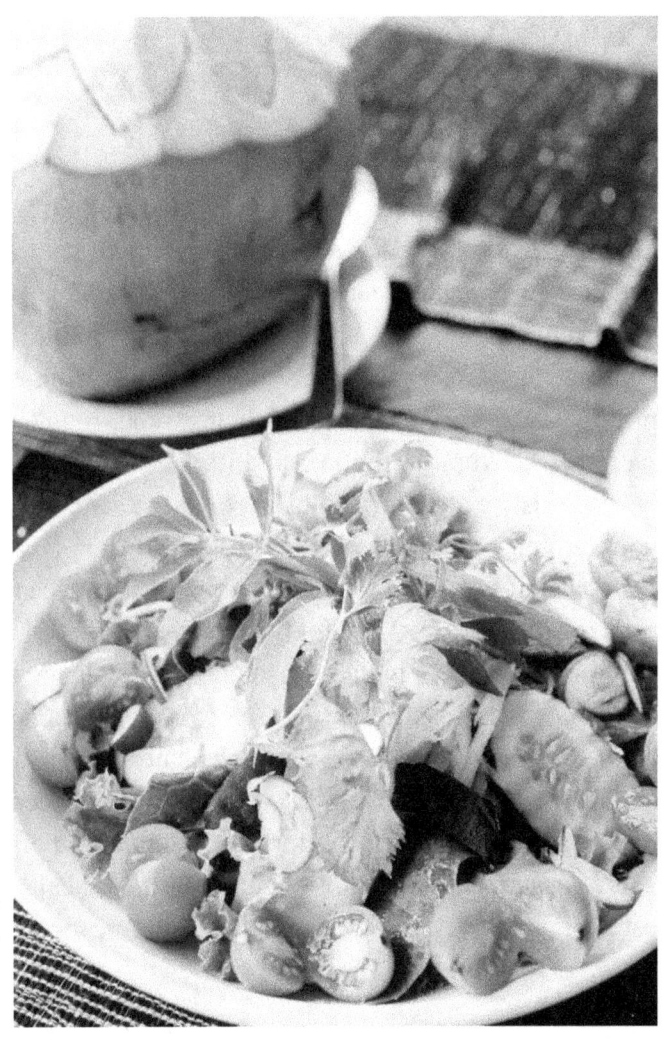

Chapter 15: Moving Forward

Sustaining an Anti-Cancer Lifestyle

Living an anti-cancer lifestyle involves ongoing commitment and proactive steps to maintain health and prevent cancer recurrence. It's about making consistent choices that support your body's natural defences against cancer, including dietary habits, physical activity, mental well-being, and regular medical checkups. Adopting an anti-cancer lifestyle is not just a temporary change but a lifelong commitment to health and wellness. It involves understanding and implementing habits that can reduce the risk of cancer and support overall well-being. Key aspects include maintaining a balanced diet rich in anti-cancer nutrients, staying physically active, managing stress, ensuring adequate sleep, and staying informed about the latest research in cancer prevention. This holistic approach combines diet, exercise, mental health, and regular health screenings to create a robust defence against cancer.

1. **Balanced Diet:** A diet rich in fruits, vegetables, whole grains, and lean proteins provides essential nutrients that can help prevent cancer.

Implementation: Incorporate a variety of colourful fruits and vegetables, whole grains, and lean proteins into your meals. Focus on plant-based foods that are high in fibre and antioxidants.

2. Regular Physical Activity: Regular exercise can help maintain a healthy weight, reduce inflammation, and boost the immune system.

Implementation: Aim for at least 150 minutes of moderate aerobic activity or 75 minutes of vigorous activity each week, along with strength training exercises twice a week.

3. Stress Management: Chronic stress can weaken the immune system and increase the risk of cancer.

Implementation: Practise stress-reducing techniques such as yoga, meditation, deep breathing exercises, and hobbies that you enjoy.

4. Adequate Sleep: Quality sleep is essential for immune function, hormone balance, and overall health.

Implementation: Aim for 7-9 hours of sleep per night. Establish a regular sleep schedule and create a restful sleep environment.

5. Avoiding Harmful Substances: Limiting exposure to carcinogens such as tobacco, excessive alcohol, and environmental toxins is crucial for cancer prevention.

Implementation: Avoid smoking, limit alcohol intake to moderate levels, and be mindful of environmental exposures by using natural cleaning products and avoiding processed foods with harmful additives.

6. Maintaining a Healthy Weight: Obesity is a risk factor for several types of cancer.

Implementation: Combine a balanced diet with regular exercise to maintain a healthy weight. Monitor your body mass index (BMI) and adjust your lifestyle as needed.

7. Staying Informed: Staying updated on the latest research and recommendations can help you make informed decisions about your health.

Implementation: Read reputable sources of health information, attend health seminars, and participate in support groups for cancer prevention.

8. Building a Support Syste: Emotional support from family, friends, and support groups can improve mental health and adherence to healthy habits.

Implementation: Engage with a community of like-minded individuals who are committed to an anti-cancer lifestyle. Share experiences and support each other.

9. Mindful Eating: Paying attention to what and how you eat can improve digestion and nutrient absorption.
Implementation: Practise mindful eating by savouring your food, eating slowly, and paying attention to hunger and fullness cues.

10. Hydration: Proper hydration supports all bodily functions, including detoxification and nutrient transport.
Implementation: Drink plenty of water throughout the day. Limit sugary drinks and opt for water, herbal teas, and natural fruit juices.

11. Limit Sugar and Processed Foods
Excess sugar and processed foods can lead to obesity and increased cancer risk.
Implementation: Reduce your intake of sugary snacks, sodas, and processed foods. Choose whole, natural foods whenever possible.

12. Positive Mental Attitude: A positive outlook can enhance your immune function and improve overall health.
Implementation: Cultivate a positive mental attitude through practices such as gratitude, positive

affirmations, and surrounding yourself with positive influences.

Continuous Learning and Adaptation

Adopting and maintaining an anti-cancer lifestyle requires a commitment to continuous learning and the ability to adapt to new information and changing circumstances. This approach ensures that you stay informed about the latest research, nutritional guidelines, and health practices that can help prevent cancer and promote overall well-being. Continuous learning and adaptation involve staying curious and proactive about your health. It means regularly updating your knowledge about cancer prevention, understanding how new research findings can impact your lifestyle, and being flexible in implementing changes to your diet, exercise routines, and other health habits. This dynamic approach allows you to make informed decisions, improve your health practices over time, and respond effectively to new challenges.

1. Staying Informed: Keeping up with the latest research helps you stay ahead in cancer prevention.
Implementation: Regularly read scientific journals, health magazines, and reputable online sources to

stay updated on new findings in cancer research and prevention.

2. Attending Workshops and Seminars: Participating in educational events can provide in-depth knowledge and practical tips. **Implementation:** Attend local or online workshops, seminars, and conferences focused on nutrition, cancer prevention, and healthy living.

3. Reading Books and Articles: Books and articles can offer comprehensive insights into specific topics. **implementation:** Read books by experts in nutrition and cancer prevention, and subscribe to health magazines or online platforms that provide regular updates and articles.

4. Participating in Support Groups: Support groups offer shared experiences and collective wisdom. **Implementation:** Join support groups or online forums where you can exchange information, tips, and experiences with others who are committed to an anti-cancer lifestyle.

5. Consulting Healthcare Professionals: Healthcare professionals can provide personalised advice based on the latest research.

Implementation: Regularly consult with your doctor, nutritionist, or oncologist to get professional advice tailored to your health needs.

6. **Adapting Diet Based on New Research:** Nutritional guidelines can change as new evidence emerges.

Implementation: Stay flexible with your diet, incorporating new foods and practices that are shown to have cancer-fighting properties as recommended by recent studies.

7. **Incorporating New Exercise Regimens:** Exercise recommendations can evolve based on new health insights.

Implementation: Update your exercise routine based on the latest fitness research, trying new activities that can boost your health and prevent cancer.

8. **Embracing Technology:** Technology can enhance your ability to learn and adapt.

Implementation: Use apps and online tools for tracking your diet, exercise, and health metrics. Follow health blogs and podcasts for the latest tips and trends.

9. **Being Open to Change:** Flexibility allows you to incorporate beneficial changes into your lifestyle.

Implementation: Cultivate an open mindset towards changing habits and trying new approaches that may better support your health.

10. **Continuous Education:** Education is a lifelong process that supports sustained health.

Implementation: Enrol in online courses or certifications related to nutrition, health, and cancer prevention to deepen your knowledge.

11. **Seeking Diverse Sources of Information:** Different sources offer varied perspectives and insights.

Implementation: Read from a variety of sources including academic journals, health websites, and books by different authors to get a well-rounded understanding.

12. **Regular Health Check-Ups:** Regular medical check-ups help in early detection and prevention.

Implementation: Schedule regular visits to your healthcare provider to monitor your health status and get updated advice based on your current condition.

Building a Support System

Building a robust support system is essential for anyone navigating the challenges of cancer prevention or recovery. This system includes a network of family, friends, healthcare professionals, and support groups that provide emotional, practical, and informational assistance. Having a strong support system enhances your resilience, provides comfort during tough times, and ensures you have access to the resources you need for maintaining an anti-cancer lifestyle. A well-rounded support system offers a multi-faceted approach to cancer prevention and recovery. It includes emotional support from loved ones, practical help with daily tasks, professional guidance from healthcare providers, and the shared experiences of support groups. This collective network helps you stay motivated, reduces feelings of isolation, and provides various perspectives and solutions to the challenges you face.

1. Emotional Support from Family and Friends: Emotional backing from loved ones helps you cope with stress and maintain a positive outlook.
Implementation: Communicate openly with your family and friends about your journey and lean on them for emotional support.

2. Practical Assistance: Help with everyday tasks can reduce your stress and allow you to focus on your health.
Implementation: Delegate chores and responsibilities to family members or friends willing to assist with cooking, cleaning, or running errands.

3. Professional Guidance: Healthcare professionals provide expert advice and treatment plans.
Implementation: Regularly consult with your doctors, nutritionists, and therapists to get professional guidance tailored to your needs.

4. Joining Support Group: Support groups offer shared experiences and a sense of community.
Implementation: Join local or online support groups where you can share your journey, exchange tips, and receive encouragement from others in similar situations.

5. Access to Resources: A support system connects you to valuable resources and information.
Implementation: Utilise the resources provided by your support network, including books, websites, and community services.

6. Building a Communication Network: Effective communication keeps your support system cohesive and responsive.
Implementation: Use communication tools like group chats, social media, or regular meetings to keep everyone in your support network informed and engaged.

7. Emotional and Mental Health Support: Mental health is crucial for overall well-being and resilience.
Implementation: Seek counselling or therapy to address emotional challenges and develop coping strategies.

8. Educational Workshops and Seminars: Education empowers you with knowledge and skills.
Implementation: Attend workshops, seminars, and webinars on cancer prevention, nutrition, and wellness to stay informed and motivated.

9. Engaging in Community Activities: Community involvement offers additional support and social interaction.
Implementation: Participate in community events, volunteer work, or local health initiatives to expand your support network and stay active.

10. Financial and Legal Support: Financial stability and legal advice are crucial during health challenges.
Implementation: Seek help from financial advisors, social workers, or legal experts to manage expenses and navigate insurance or legal issues.

11. Creating a Positive Environment: A positive environment boosts mental and emotional well-being.

Implementation: Surround yourself with supportive, positive individuals and create a home environment that promotes relaxation and wellness.

12. Utilising Online Resources: Online resources provide easy access to information and support.

Implementation: Explore reputable online forums, websites, and social media groups dedicated to cancer prevention and healthy living.

Final Thoughts and Encouragement

As you embark on your journey towards a healthier, anti-cancer lifestyle, remember that every step you take matters. While the road ahead may seem daunting at times, know that you are not alone. With dedication, resilience, and the support of your loved ones, you can overcome obstacles and make meaningful changes that promote your well-being and reduce your risk of cancer. In the pursuit of a lifestyle that combats cancer, it's essential to maintain a positive mindset and draw strength from within. Reflect on your motivations, set realistic goals, and celebrate your progress, no matter how small. Surround yourself with a supportive network of family, friends, and healthcare professionals who uplift and encourage you along the way. Remember that change takes time, and each decision you make towards a healthier lifestyle is a step in the right direction.

1. **Embrace Progress, Not Perfection:** ecognize that adopting a healthier lifestyle is a journey, not a destination. Focus on making gradual changes and celebrate each milestone you achieve.

2. **Stay Motivated:** Keep your reasons for pursuing an anti-cancer lifestyle at the forefront of your mind. Whether it's for yourself, your loved ones, or future generations, let your motivation drive your commitment to change.

3. **Practice Self-Compassion:** Be kind to yourself on this journey. Accept that setbacks may occur, but use them as opportunities for growth and learning rather than reasons for discouragement.

4. **Find Joy in the Process:** Explore new recipes, activities, and experiences that bring you joy and enhance your well-being. Cultivate a sense of enjoyment in living a healthy lifestyle.

5. **Lean on Your Support System:** Don't hesitate to reach out to your support network when you need encouragement or assistance. Share your successes and challenges with those who uplift and inspire you.

6. Stay Educated: Continue to educate yourself about cancer prevention, nutrition, and overall health. Knowledge empowers you to make informed decisions and navigate your journey with confidence.

7. Practice Gratitude: Take a moment each day to express gratitude for the blessings in your life, including your health, relationships, and opportunities for growth.

8. Celebrate Your Achievements: Acknowledge and celebrate your accomplishments, no matter how small. Each healthy choice you make contributes to your overall well-being and deserves recognition.

9. Visualise Your Future: Envision the vibrant, healthy life you aspire to live. Use this vision as motivation to stay committed to your journey and overcome obstacles along the way.

10. Spread Positivity: Share your experiences and insights with others who may benefit from your journey. Your story has the power to inspire and encourage those facing similar challenges.

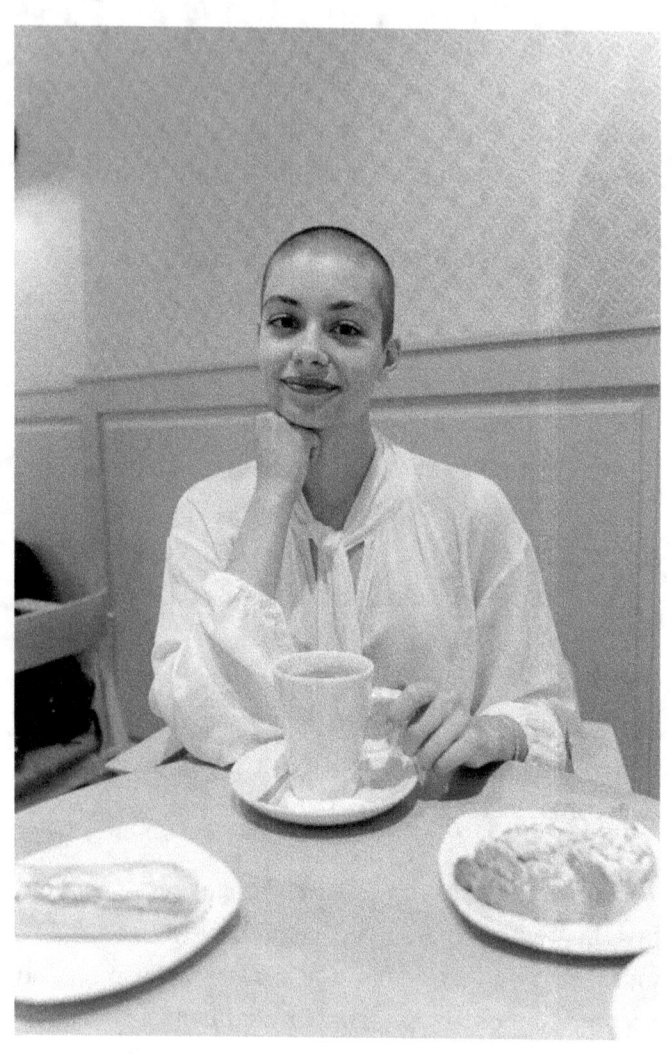

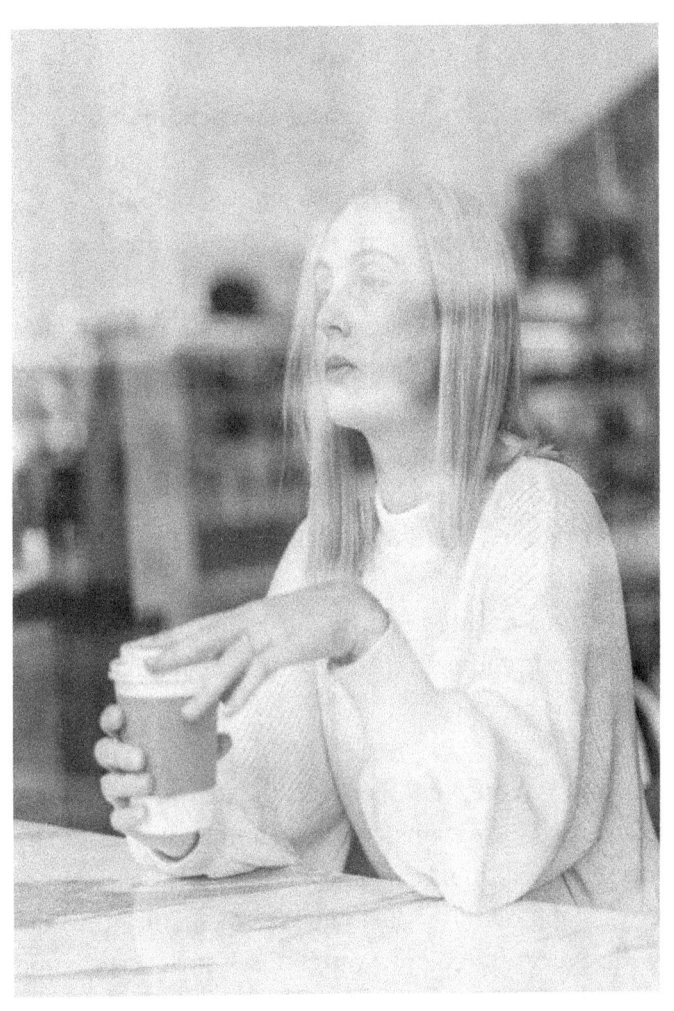

CONCLUSION

Beat Cancer, The Anti-Cancer Kitchen, invite you to unlock the potential of your kitchen as a fortress against cancer. This isn't just a cookbook, it's a blueprint for empowerment and transformation. By harnessing the synergies of diet, fight, and plant-based nutrition, you are stepping into a world where every meal becomes a strategic strike against cancer.

Picture this, your kitchen, a battleground where you wield the weapons of delicious, simple, and anti-cancer recipes. Each dish you create is a testament to your commitment to wellness and vitality. With every bite, you are not just nourishing your body; you are arming yourself with the tools to combat cancer head-on.

As you savour the flavours and textures of your plant-based creations, remember that you hold the key to a healthier, cancer-free future. Your journey doesn't end with the last page of this book; it begins with every ingredient you choose and every recipe you master. This is your chance to take control, to fight back, and to emerge victorious in the battle against cancer.

So, let your kitchen be your battlefield, your recipes your weapons, and your determination your driving force. Transform your kitchen into a powerhouse of anti-cancer goodness, and let every meal you prepare be a step towards a brighter, healthier tomorrow. Embrace the power of your plate and join the fight against cancer today.

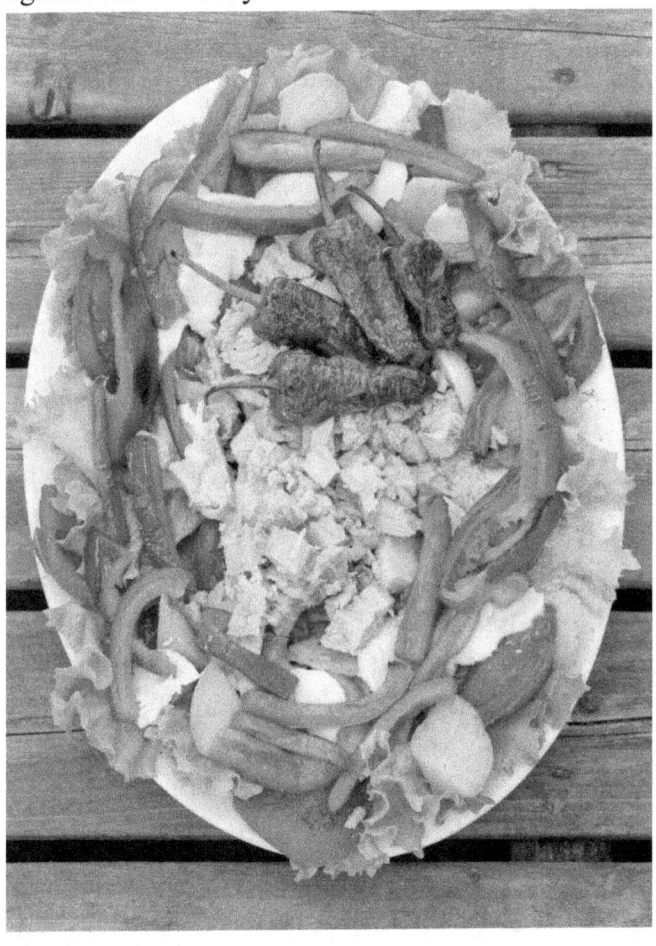

Free special Bonus for you

Discover the life-changing benefits of "Beat Cancer, The Anti Cancer Kitchen" and transform your culinary space into a powerful ally against cancer. As a special token of my appreciation, I am offering an exclusive bonus just for you! Unlock a treasure trove of additional resources, expert tips, and mouth-watering recipes designed to supercharge your journey towards optimal health. This free bonus is my way of saying "thank you" for taking the first step in prioritising your well-being and joining me in the fight against cancer. Don't miss out on this extraordinary opportunity to enhance your kitchen's cancer-fighting potential. Claim your free special bonus today and embark on a flavorful, health-conscious adventure that nourishes both body and soul!

Anti-Cancer Recipes Index

The Anti-Cancer Recipes Index is a diverse collection of delicious, health-boosting recipes created to support individuals in their journey towards optimal well-being. This extensive index caters to a wide range of dietary preferences and needs, making it the perfect resource for anyone looking to transform their kitchen into a powerful ally against cancer.

1. Variety of Recipes: The Anti-Cancer Recipes Index offers a vast array of recipes that cater to different dietary preferences, ensuring there's something for everyone, whether you're vegetarian, vegan, or gluten-free. This variety makes it easy to find meals that suit your specific needs while still being delicious and nutritious.

2. Cancer-Fighting Ingredients: Each recipe in the index contains essential nutrients that have been shown to promote overall health and well-being, helping to reduce the risk of cancer and other chronic diseases. By incorporating these ingredients into your meals, you're taking a proactive approach to your health.

3. Expert Guidance: The recipes in the index have been crafted by experienced chefs and nutritionists who understand the importance of maintaining good health through proper nutrition. Their expertise ensures that each dish not only tastes great but also supports your well-being.

4. Easy-to-Follow Instructions: Every recipe in the index comes with clear, step-by-step instructions that make meal preparation a breeze, even for those with limited cooking experience. This allows you to create delicious, healthy dishes without the stress.

5. Time-Saving Tips: In addition to easy instructions, the index provides helpful tips and techniques for making meal preparation more efficient, so you can spend less time in the kitchen and more time enjoying your food.

6. Delicious Flavors: Contrary to popular belief, healthy eating doesn't have to be boring or bland. The recipes in the index are packed with flavour, proving that nutritious meals can also be a delight for your taste buds.

7. Inspiration for Mealtime Variety: With a wide range of creative and unique recipe ideas, the Anti-Cancer Recipes Index ensures that you'll never be bored with your meals. Say goodbye to mealtime monotony and hello to exciting new flavours and combinations.

8. Proactive Health Approach: By incorporating cancer-fighting ingredients into your diet, you're taking a preventative approach to your health and well-being. This proactive mindset can have lasting benefits for your overall quality of life.

9. Holistic Health Support: The recipes in the index don't just nourish your body; they also support your mental and emotional well-being. By providing a foundation for overall health, these meals can contribute to a happier, more balanced life.

10. Accessible for All: Whether you're a seasoned cook or a complete novice, the Anti-Cancer Recipes Index is designed to be accessible and user-friendly. Everyone can benefit from these delicious, health-boosting meals, regardless of their skill level in the kitchen.

Glossary of Terms

Glossary of terms tailored specifically for the book title, "BEAT CANCER, THE ANTI CANCER KITCHEN, Transforming Your Kitchen Into A Weapon Against Cancer

1. Anti-Cancer Lifestyle: A way of living that focuses on daily habits and practices to reduce cancer risk and promote overall well-being. Living an anti-cancer lifestyle involves adopting healthy habits such as eating a nutritious diet, staying physically active, managing stress, and avoiding harmful substances like tobacco. By prioritising these practices, individuals can help lower their risk of developing cancer and improve their overall quality of life.

2. Phytochemicals: Naturally occurring compounds found in plants that have potential health benefits, including reducing inflammation and preventing cancer cell growth. Phytochemicals are compounds that give plants their unique colours, flavours, and aromas. Some common examples include lycopene in tomatoes, resveratrol in grapes, and sulforaphane in broccoli. These compounds have been studied for their potential role in reducing inflammation and preventing the growth of cancer cells.

3. Inflammation: The body's response to injury or infection, which can sometimes contribute to cancer development when chronic or excessive. Inflammation is a natural immune response that helps protect the body from harm. However, chronic inflammation can increase the risk of cancer and other diseases. Some factors that contribute to chronic inflammation include poor diet, lack of exercise, stress, and exposure to environmental toxins.

4. Oxidative Stress: An imbalance between free radicals and antioxidants in the body, leading to potential cell damage and increasing cancer risk. Oxidative stress occurs when there are more free radicals in the body than antioxidants to neutralise them. This imbalance can cause damage to cells and DNA, potentially increasing the risk of cancer. Reducing exposure to environmental toxins, consuming a diet rich in antioxidants, and engaging in regular physical activity can help manage oxidative stress.

5. Immune System: The body's defence mechanism against diseases, including cancer. A strong immune system can help prevent cancer development. The immune system is composed of various cells, tissues, and organs that work together to protect the body from infections and diseases. Maintaining a healthy immune system through proper nutrition, regular exercise, adequate sleep, and stress management can help reduce the risk of cancer.

6. Whole Grains: Grains that contain all parts of the grain kernel, providing essential nutrients and potential cancer-fighting compounds. Whole grains, such as brown rice, quinoa, and oats, are rich in fibre, vitamins, minerals, and phytochemicals. Consuming whole grains instead of refined grains can help improve digestion, regulate blood sugar, and potentially reduce the risk of certain cancers.

7. Cruciferous Vegetables: A family of vegetables, including broccoli and kale, that contain compounds known for their potential anti-cancer properties. Cruciferous vegetables are rich in vitamins, minerals, fibre, and phytochemicals. Some examples include broccoli, kale, cauliflower, and Brussels sprouts. These vegetables have been studied for their potential role in preventing cancer cell growth and reducing inflammation.

8. Meal Planning: The process of organising and arranging meals in advance to ensure a balanced, healthy diet. Meal planning involves deciding what foods to eat and when, based on individual preferences and dietary requirements. This practice can help individuals make healthier food choices, save time and money, and reduce stress related to meal preparation.

9. Meal Prep: The act of preparing or partially preparing meals in advance to save time and encourage healthier eating choices throughout the week. Meal prep can involve cooking large batches of food and portioning them into individual servings, pre-chopping vegetables, or marinating proteins. By dedicating time to meal prep, individuals can make healthier choices throughout the week and avoid relying on unhealthy convenience foods.

9. Mindful Eating: A practice that involves focusing on the present moment and paying attention to the sensations and emotions associated with eating. Mindful eating encourages individuals to savour their food, eat slowly, and listen to their body's hunger and fullness cues. This practice can improve digestion, promote portion control, and enhance the overall enjoyment of meals.

Resources and References

Here are ten websites providing valuable information and resources on cancer prevention through diet and lifestyle.

1. American Institute for Cancer Research (AICR) - https://www.aicr.org/. A leading organisation focused on cancer prevention through diet, physical activity, and maintaining a healthy weight.

2. World Cancer Research Fund International (WCRF) - https://www.wcrf.org/. Provides evidence-based information on cancer prevention, including diet and lifestyle recommendations.

3. Cancer.Net https://www.cancer.net/. A patient-oriented website with information on various types of cancer, treatment, and prevention.

4. National Cancer Institute (NCI) - https://www.cancer.gov/ Offers comprehensive information on cancer research, prevention, and treatment options.

5. American Cancer Society (ACS) - https://www.cancer.org/. Provides information on various types of cancer, treatments, and healthy lifestyle practices for cancer prevention.

6. Cancer Research UK - https://www.cancerresearchuk.org/. A UK-based organisation providing information on cancer prevention, treatment, and research.

7. Memorial Sloan Kettering Cancer Center - https://www.mskcc.org/. A leading cancer centre offering resources on cancer prevention, treatment, and support.

8. Harvard T.H. Chan School of Public Health - https://www.hsph.harvard.edu/. Provides information on public health topics, including cancer prevention through diet and lifestyle.

9. Johns Hopkins Medicine - https://www.hopkinsmedicine.org/

9. The University of Texas MD Anderson Cancer Center - https://www.mdanderson.org/ These websites offer reliable and up-to-date information on cancer prevention and healthy living practices. Explore them to learn more about how a healthy lifestyle can reduce the risk of developing cancer.

Acknowledgments

Acknowledgements for "BEAT CANCER, THE ANTI CANCER KITCHEN, Transforming Your Kitchen Into A Weapon Against Cancer" by Raquel, a cancer survivor.

As a cancer survivor and the author of this book, I am incredibly grateful to the numerous individuals who have supported and inspired me throughout my journey.

First and foremost, I want to thank my healthcare team for their unwavering dedication and expertise in guiding me through my cancer treatment and recovery. Their compassion and skill have been invaluable in my fight against cancer.

I am also deeply appreciative of the researchers, scientists, and healthcare professionals who have devoted their lives to understanding cancer prevention through diet and lifestyle. Their discoveries and insights have laid the groundwork for the information shared within these pages.

To the nutritionists, chefs, and home cooks who have shared their knowledge and creativity in developing cancer-fighting recipes, I extend my sincere gratitude. Your expertise and passion for healthy living have been instrumental in demonstrating that a nutritious lifestyle can be both practical and enjoyable.

To my family, friends, and colleagues, thank you for your endless support, encouragement, and personal stories that have motivated me to create this resource.

23 cancer-fighting ingredients
1. Broccoli
2. Garlic
3. Turmeric
4. Green tea
5. Blueberries
6. Salmon
7. Tomatoes
8. Spinach
9. Kale
10. Quinoa
11. Chia seeds
12. Beans and legumes
13. Avocado

14. Sweet potatoes
15. Walnuts
16. Flaxseeds
17. Pomegranate
18. Olive oil
19. Cruciferous vegetables (cauliflower, Brussels sprouts)
20. Berries (strawberries, raspberries, blackberries)
21. Ginger
22. Citrus fruits (oranges, lemons, grapefruit)
23. Onions

These ingredients contain powerful compounds and antioxidants that have been linked to cancer prevention and overall health benefits. Remember that a balanced diet with a variety of whole, nutrient-dense foods is essential for maintaining good health and reducing the risk of chronic diseases like cancer.

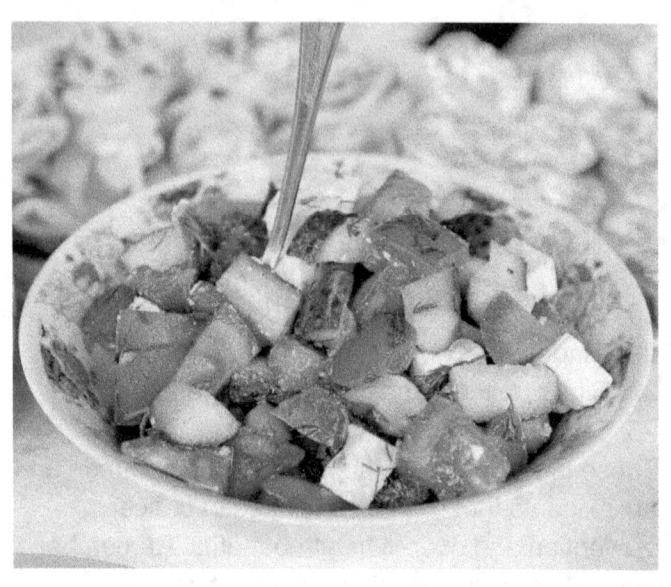

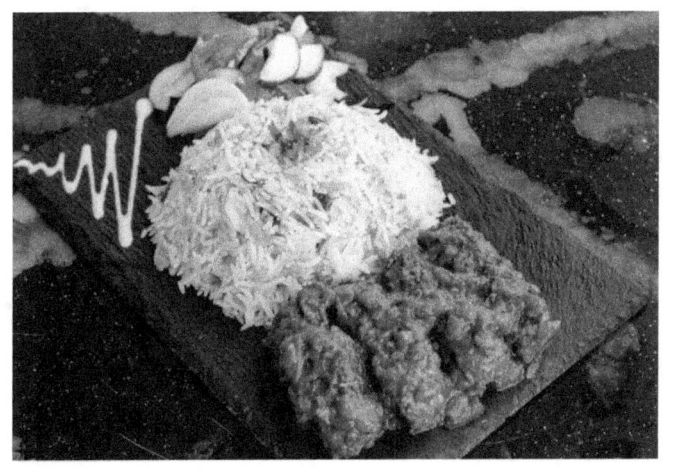